Overcoming Church Hurt & Abuse

Freedom from Past Hurts.
Freedom to Soar.

Erin Lamb

Overcoming Church Hurt & Abuse
Published by Lamb Enterprises LLC
Dublin, Ohio 43016
Https://www.empowered-free.com

Jacket Design: Prudence Mukhura
ISBN-13: 978-0-578-53953-9

Dedication

To every person who has been told to build a bridge and just get over what you have suffered, this is for you. May you find healing, hope, and restoration.

Acknowledgements

I would love to specifically offer a special thanks to the following people:

All the brave clients I have seen over the years. Thank you for sharing your stories, your hearts, and trusting me to walk with you on this journey of freedom.

My parents who continued to tell me I could do and be anything. Thank you for believing in me and the vision to positively impact the world.

Dr. Scott Bitcon who gave up hours of his time to train, teach, and mentor in the area of deep inner healing. Thank you!

Madaline Sanders and Jarmila Gordon for editing this book.

And to friends and those who have encouraged writing and continuation of the pursuit of healing and justice in our world.

Table of Contents

Foreword

First, thank you for picking up this book. I am thinking of you and hope your life is transformed in a positive way. With every chapter, I hope the layers of pain are peeled back, soothed, and the hurt lessens. We were not created for a lifetime of pain and suffering. You may be suffering from memories that haunt you. There may be a few of you who have turned your back on God all together. If God is so good, how could He allow such pain and suffering? If God is so good, why are some of His supposed "children" more like the devil than Jesus in their behavior? Keep reading, I address questions similar to these, and more.

Why write a book about overcoming church hurt and abuse? This book was not on the list of books in queue. It sprung up out of my spirit in response to things I see in sessions with abused individuals. I have training in using faith-based tools, a prayer based model, to help victims of abuse and post-traumatic stress disorder (PTSD) find freedom and healing. I have spent the past few years teaching others how to help abuse victims and have years of experience using faith based methods with victims.

This book was also birthed out of response to abuse from clergy exposed in the media. I have encountered numerous people in my life who have simply given up on church, on God, and at the root is church hurt. There was a person or more than one person who hurt them severely and they did not recover. Maybe they were shunned by the church because they sinned or would not conform to a certain pattern of thought. Maybe they were never welcomed in the church. Maybe they trusted their child with a person at the church and later found out the person they trusted was an abuser.

How do we navigate through the hard things that happen in communities of faith? There are people who are told to simply forgive and forget. There are people who are told to build a bridge and simply get over what happened to them. Some are quoted the scripture, "…forgetting those things which are behind and reaching forward to those things which are ahead (Philippians 3:13b)." Pretending the negative things that happen in communities of faith have not occurred is detrimental to everyone. We do not heal what is ignored, avoided, or denied.

If I have a major injury to my body, it does not just heal on its own. We would probably advise a person who was just run over by a ten-ton truck, if they even survived, to forgo trying to run a marathon. We can see physical injury; therefore, there is greater attention to those wounds. Wounds in the soul are just as important. I have concern for those who pretend they have not been injured and wounded in their soul. Additionally, I have concern for those who encourage others to pretend they have not been wounded or damaged.

There are times when the attempts to be merciful actually violate justice or godly accountability. If we are truly people of faith, we believe in the healing power of forgiveness. Forgiveness is not always what people think it is. We cover forgiveness as well in one of the chapters.

I have spent years studying the soul (mind, will, emotions) and how the soul heals. It is not as simple as forgive and forget as we are told so many times in communities of faith. It's also not a pull yourself up by your bootstraps because *greater is He who is in you than He who is in the world*. I have heard various insensitive things in my own journey with God from people who claim to know God. I have heard these same comments from some of the people who are struggling.

The things we bury do not heal; they show up later. Buried pain can crack our lenses and shift our perspective. If one pastor abuses children, there can be a tainted view of all clergy. The wounds that are not healed scream out in the midnight hours or in moments when a memory is triggered.

My hope for Overcoming Church Hurt & Abuse, is for people to find wholeness and healing in Jesus. I am sorry if you have been wounded by a professing Christian. I am sorry if your experiences shifted your perception of God. Jesus is not an abuser, nor does He condone abuse. Love is the highest objective of God. If what has been presented to you is abuse, control, manipulation, or oppression, it violates the expression of the heart of Jesus.

Please know I am praying for you. I want you to walk in total and complete freedom. Freedom is the objective. No person is free who carries the wounds and buried negative emotions of the past. It is time to unpack the baggage, empty out the heaviness, and invite healing into our souls. We cannot change what has been done to us. We can step into a new beginning together. We can pursue wholeness together. God desires your wholeness, too!

Introduction

We were created by love (God), to be loved, then to love.

There is no part of genuine love that involves abuse. I know there are people who misquote the Bible and misinterpret the text to promote the mistreatment of human beings. People wrongly used the Bible to promote slavery in parts of the United States. There are still people in parts of the world using the Bible to abuse, oppress, and silence women.

I often wonder if people pay attention to the words and lifestyle of Jesus. He stated so plainly that His disciples, true followers, would be known by their agape love (sacrificial, unselfish, and pure love) (John 13:34-35). Jesus stated so plainly that His mission was to reveal the heart of the Father. If we want to know the heart of the Father, we can look to Jesus as a pure representation. According to the Bible. "If anyone says, 'I love God,' and hates (works against) his [Christian] brother he is a liar; for the one who does not love his brother whom he has seen, cannot love God whom he has not seen,"-1 John 4:20 (AMP). Along with this verse we are told in Romans that love fulfills the law because love does no harm to its neighbor (Romans 13:10).

We see in the person of Jesus a man who loved with His entire life. The love that flowed through Jesus of Nazareth was transformative love. It was and is a love saturated in humility and overflowing with goodness. We see in the person of Jesus a person willing to stoop down low in order to lift others up. We see a loving servant who chose to humbly serve instead of bark out orders. We see purity in Jesus, in His actions and treatment of people. We do not see a bully, controller, abuser, nor do we see Jesus seeking to degrade women. We see love.

God is love. You and I were created by love (God), to be loved, then to love.

"Beloved, let us [unselfishly] love and seek the best for one another, for love is from God; and everyone who loves [others] is born of God and knows God [through personal experience]. The one who *does not love* has not become acquainted with God [does not and never did know Him], for God is love. [He is the originator of love, and it is an enduring attribute of His nature.]"-1 John 4:7-8 (AMP).

Abuse and mistreatment are not love. Love seeks what is best for the other person. Love is not selfish. Love is not proud. Love is not driven by ego. Love is not lustful nor greedy. Love does not take advantage, nor is love a consumer. Love is not perverted. Love is not harmful. Love protects. Love is not a predator. Love collaborates with others. Love is the highest aim of God. Those who claim to know God and fail to love, do not know God. It is possible to know the Bible and **not** know God. The Pharisees could quote the law, but they did not know God.

In my years of working with abuse victims, there is a common theme of a person distorting love, shifting of the person's perspective of who they are and in many instances developing a distorted view of God. It can be even more damaging when the abuser claims to be speaking for God, representing God, or is in a position of authority. There are people who believe that professing to be a Christian, or holding a position in a church means that person is safe and loving. This is not always the case.

My hopes for writing this short book are that people who have been greatly wounded by the behaviors of professing Christians can find freedom: freedom from hurt, freedom from offense, freedom from mistrust of clergy or leaders, and freedom from trauma.

Let's dive into God's heart together and overcome with Jesus. You and I were created to be loved, to know love, and then to love.

Chapter 1

Where is Jesus?

Jesus=God With Us

"As the Father has loved me, so have I loved you", - Jesus Christ (John 15:9).

I have spent a good chunk of my ministry time dealing with people who have been severely wounded. I have been trained in prayer ministry, soaking prayer, deep inner healing, and deliverance (overcoming spiritual oppression). I have years of experience dealing with abuse victims either from churches or off the street. I have heard every manner of horror story, and I often wish I could forget the stories. When you add in recent work with victims of human trafficking, it compounds the horror stories. There are children as young as 2 years old that are being abused. I am stunned by the stories and moved by the intensity of their pain.

I have experienced personally gross mistreatment by people who claimed to be Christians or were clergy. I have not been sexually abused, yet I understand what it is like to trust another Christian and have them betray that trust. When they claim to be a person who loves God, it can be confusing. If God is love, the person claims to know God, then why is their behavior unloving or abusive?

One of the things I believe we need to address is how do we heal? How do we have the tough conversations about abuse and mistreatment? How do we navigate into the realms of freedom God promised? How do we move past just telling people to forgive and pretend nothing happened? As I stated earlier, there are people who believe we should just forgot those things behind us and press ahead. What happens to the person who has forgiven (to the best of their ability) and they are still suffering?

I believe the answers to those questions come from the one who promised to reveal the love of the Father to the world. We can feel forsaken and forgotten if we have suffered abuse or gross mistreatment. The truth is God was there and took no pleasure in the pain or suffering. If you have been abused, right now, I would like for you to meditate on this truth. **God was there. God hated the abuse. God weeps. God loves you.**

Your heart may scream out, "Why didn't God stop my abuser? If God is love, why didn't God do something to stop the abuse? If God is all powerful, then why didn't God stop the horror that went on and on in my life? If God is so good, why did He allow this horrible thing to occur in my life or the life of my child? If God is so good, why didn't He just strike my abuser dead or stop them from ever entering ministry?" I have heard these questions in deep inner healing sessions. I have also witnessed people struggle greatly with their concepts of God, relationship with God, and struggle with receiving the love of God because of the abuse they suffered.

I will tell you one of the most loving things God did for humanity was to provide us with free will. We, human beings, have been given this incredible opportunity to choose. Evil exists because of the **abuse of free will**. God does not create evil people. People make choices that align with evil. If God controlled us and our choices, then there would be perfection in the world. God is not a controller. God allows choice. Where there is no ability to make decisions, there is control. Certainly, there are consequences for our poor choices, and there are laws in place to help prevent evil. People can still break the law. They are not robots. God did not create robots.

Oh, how I wish at times God would hijack the will of humanity and stop human trafficking, abuse of children, wars, all gun violence, and force a kinder humanity. The truth is forcing humanity to do what God wants violates the character of God. Jesus was not forced to go to the cross. He chose to go.

The freedom to choose is a blessing when our choices and the choices of those around us align with good. This freedom to choose is detrimental when humans choose to do things that are toxic, damaging, abusive, and harmful. I heard a quote that was quite freeing for me during a time of being mistreated by Christians. The quote says, "People are normally not against you; they are primarily for themselves." Selfishness is often the root of mistreatment. When a person is more concerned for themselves than they are for others, it creates problems for everyone.

I wish I had all the answers as to why God does not prevent all harm on this planet. I do not possess all the answers. I do know that God abhors abuse and does not take delight in our unjust suffering. Jesus suffered for the sins of humanity. It was not frivolous suffering. There are millions of people suffering on this planet, and that is not a representation of God's heart for humanity.

Jesus stated, "...I came that they may have and enjoy life, and have it in abundance [to the full, till it overflows]," - (John 10:10b AMP). Abuse is not living life to the fullest. It is not life abundantly. Abuse is not freedom. I have not met a person being abused who was free. I have not encountered an abused person who was truly loved by their abuser. Abuse is not love; it is void of Jesus.

For a moment, ponder the mission statement of Jesus out of Luke 4:18-19 (AMP).

"The Spirit of the Lord is upon Me (the Messiah), because He has anointed Me to preach the good news to the poor. He has sent Me to announce release (pardon, forgiveness) to the captives, and recovery of sight to the blind, to set free those who are oppressed (downtrodden, bruised, crushed by tragedy) to proclaim the favorable year of the Lord [the day when salvation and the favor of God abound greatly]."

Jesus came for **FREEDOM from oppression**! Love came down to bring freedom, not bondage. Love came down to bring healing. Love came down to be with us. After His ascension, the Spirit of God became the seeker of mankind to dwell within those who believe. From the beginning of time, God has been pursuing a loving relationship with humanity. This relationship, as stated before, is based on love and freedom from evil.

Jesus hates when we are abused. It is not the nature of His heart to enjoy mistreatment, abuse, bullying, or the pain of any person. One of the most comforting things people experience in deep inner healing sessions is God revealing His truth about what happened to them. God is invited into the painful memories. I had a lady who always believed that God did not love her because He did not stop her abuse from occurring. During the recall of the memory, I simply asked God to reveal His truth about what happened to her. She saw a picture of Jesus preventing her abuse from being worse than it was, pulling her abuser off her.

People misunderstand the Father's heart towards the abuse and mistreatment of Jesus. God knew that the sacrifice of Jesus would bring freedom to so many people. Sin is the reason Jesus was crucified, not because the Father is sadistic. Misunderstanding scripture, which we will cover in a future chapter, has created platforms for many people to be abusive. There are those who believe that their suffering is somehow making them more like God. It is a misunderstanding of scripture and the heart of God. How can it bring God glory for His children to walk around wounded? If a natural parent stated, "I am going to subject you to severe abuse to teach you to be a great person," we would have the person arrested. There are people who think God is a child abuser because they do not fully understand the heart of God.

It is imperative we know the heart of God. It is also imperative we know that God is not the author of abuse. Sin is the author of abuse. Sin brings punishment and eventual death. There are people who have chosen a path of harming others and their conscious has deadened. They do not feel remorse. They do not feel love. God does not delight that there are millions of people who are being abused on this planet. God's eyes are not blind to injustice nor the cries of the oppressed. God sees. God hears. God is the just judge who will make all things right.

Jesus, Emmanuel, is God with us. God with us when life is good. God with us when life is beyond challenging. Jesus weeps over the pain that sin causes. Abuse is iniquity. It violates the very teachings of Jesus. He commanded His followers to love. Whether your experiences are recent or in the past, **God mourned with you**. God did not turn a blind eye. God loved you then and loves you today. God is one whisper or thought away longing to take away the pain, the hurt, the trauma, the horror stories that replay over and over. God is here.

One of the greatest encouragements I can offer aside from God hates that you were abused or anyone you love, is God longs to mend all the broken and hurting places. God wants to take all the pain and trade beauty for ashes. I can say this from doing years of soul healing with people and by my experiences with God. No matter how deep the cut, or how painful the experience, God longs to heal.

Maybe your anger and hurt is directed towards God. If that's the case, understand that God can handle the pain, anger, and mis-understandings. Maybe you feel abandoned or forsaken by God. Stuffing it or placing on a fake Christian mask of, "God is good all the time," while you are seething inside does not facilitate healing. I encourage people to be honest with themselves and God. God already knows the depths of your emotions and the pain. If you are angry with God, stuffing the negative emotions and pretending to be okay is not the way to find freedom. If you are angry with the church, God already knows.

There have been clients in sessions with me who found free-dom in honesty. They were honest for the first time about their feelings about what happened to them. They were honest about the hatred towards the person who abused them. They were hon-est about the shame and self-blame. Was it their fault? Could they have done something differently? Shame creates situations where people hide. There is freedom in the light. There is no freedom in hiding and pretending. It's time to stop hiding and find freedom in speaking truth.

We can see in scripture people who were transparent in their heart conditions, disappointments, and pain with God. I love King David because he was quite transparent with God. Job was trans-parent with God. Even Jesus was transparent with the Father, "Why have you forsaken me," (Matthew 27:46). Talking to God about our anger, hurt, and disappointment is a path to healing. Have you talked about it with God? Have you spoken to a safe person about what happened to you? Does anyone know or is the horror tucked away in the deep recesses of the soul?

I have dealt with people who do not believe in honest conver-sations with God. It's not my place to judge them, yet I do not at-tempt to share my inner life with them either. Wisdom comes in knowing who to talk to and who to keep on a need to know basis.

I spoke to a lady at a church once about pain I was experiencing in my relationship with God. She did not offer compassion. She was quick to tell me she never doubted God, then proceeded to look down her nose at me. I tucked my honesty back in my pocket, and I learned not to reveal any disappointment or hurt.

I learned to hide in circles of faith. I learned that pretending to be happy all the time was applauded and any sign of disappointment was quickly dismissed. I watched hurting people pretend to be on the mountain top to bypass judgement or being perceived as a weak Christian. People loved to throw scripture at me. Many were unwilling to listen and be a source of help. I recall being told by a Christian once that God was not moved by my tears, He was moved by my faith. I learned to hide pain. God taught me to release pain to Him and find healing. I was not fake or false in my expressions. I did not tell people at church about the painful things I needed to unpack with God. I am encouraging you to release pain to God and forsake hiding or false Christian happiness.

I want you to be able to express your heart to God knowing that He is on the other end listening with a heart of love. God is incredibly patient and understands what we know and what we do not know. Trying to hide pain, hurt, or anger from God is not helpful. I love that God is compassionate, slow to anger and abounding in love. This may violate your current beliefs of God or maybe what has been demonstrated to you. I can tell you from experience that God is far better than anyone has made Him out to be.

I learned through years of walking through challenging situations that God truly is love. I learned that God could handle my challenging questions, disappointments, and pain. I learned that God was not distant, unmoved, nor just watching our pain. I learned that pretending there wasn't a problem and feeling pressured to place a perpetual smile on my face was killing my soul.

My encouragement is: God can handle it all. God can handle our dialogue about what hurts, even when we think He is the author of that pain.

Have you ever been angry with God or disappointed? I will tell you that expressing what is going on in our souls can help us heal. Maybe start with a piece of paper and a note, "Where were you, God?" Maybe you were told that it's not okay to be honest with God or ask God questions. Many of the deepest wounds I have seen in sessions were with people who had deep rooted pain tied to God. It was not treated or healed. It laid inside their souls and festered. It profoundly impacted all their other relationships. What questions are you dying to ask God? What's stopping you from asking them? Maybe you will not receive the answer you want, or an answer immediately. I will tell you that God wants a relationship with you. Relationships are built on communication.

I would love for our first step to be honesty. This happened, it hurt. This happened, and I no longer choose denial. This happened, and I am (insert your negative emotion). This happened, and it impacted my views of God this way. It impacted my views of who I am this way. Can you be honest with God today?

I want you to heal. One of my greatest desires is for your heart and soul to be healed. Part of healing is getting real. We may not be able to do that with everyone. I am not recommending you go online and reveal the deepest secrets of your heart. I am encouraging starting by getting real with yourself and God. Can you start there?

Will you pray with me?

God, I do not understand all of the things you did not prevent from happening in my life. It has been painful, and I do not wish to carry this pain any longer. I am inviting you in today to show me or tell me where you were during my abuse or mistreatment. I want your truth about what happened. Today, I invite you into all the places that are wounded, even the places I have stuffed away that have not healed. Come into my heart, my soul, and make me new. I want to be healed. I want to be whole. Help me to see that you are love. You hate any mistreatment I suffered because of another person's sins. Mend me, God. Heal my heart and emotions. Remove any negative thoughts I continue to ponder because of the abuse or mistreatment. I want your thoughts. Soften any hard parts of my heart towards you. If I hold any bitterness or resentment towards you, I release it today. Help me to release all of me into your love. You are safe. My heart is safe with you. Rewrite my story so it's redemptive, and I am whole. I want to live my best life!

Activation: Grab a pen and paper. Set aside quiet time. I want you to take time to go through this exercise. Please do not skip ahead. I believe when we take our hearts to God, profound healing can occur.

1. Ask God to reveal any unhealed hurts in your heart and soul. What still hurts? What painful memory is holding you back? Write out your thoughts and memories.

2. Who created the pain? What did they do? Outline ways their behavior did not and does not match Jesus.

3. Ask God to give you His perspective of what happened. What is God's truth about what happened? Where was God?

4. What are the negative emotions attached to the memory? (Example: anger, shame, feeling dirty, resentment, pain). Ask God to take the pain away and heal all that hurts.

5. Ask God to show you any lies you came to believe because of the abuse or mistreatment. What are the lies you came to believe about God? What are the lies you came to believe about yourself? Renounce those lies. You can say, "I come out of agreement with the lie (insert the lie)."

After you work through your thoughts, feel empowered to shred, tear up, or burn those notes. My friends and I had a burn party once. All the negative things spoken over us were renounced (I am not in agreement with (insert negative statement)). We wrote down the negative things spoken over us, and then we burned the papers. A freedom proclamation was made, "I am not defined by the negative things spoken over my life!"

You are not defined by what has been done to you or said about you. You are loved! You are greatly loved!

Chapter 2

The Roots of Abuse & Misuse of the Bible

(Quoting the Bible Does Not Equal Knowing God)

"Knowing the Bible is one thing; knowing the Author is another."

It is absolutely possible to know scriptures from the Bible and not know God relationally. It is also possible to read the Bible and walk away with wrong ideas about what it says and what it means. There are people who have the wrong interpretation. How can I state such a thing? Well, when Jesus walked the earth, He encountered numerous people who knew God's law. However, they did not know God; they did not understand who Jesus was. They rejected the very person who came to represent the heart of God to the world. Not only was there a rejection of Jesus as the Son of God, there was hostility towards His message. Jesus endured abuse, and He was murdered by the ones He came to save.

An individual can quote the Bible, attend church or a temple, yet remain completely void of the likeness of God and ignorant of who God really is. As stated in the previous chapter, God is love. Those who know God will also love others. Those who do not know God, they do not love (1 John 4:8). A proclamation of knowing God is not the same as an actual relationship with God. Going to church is not the same as a personal relationship with God. We live in an age where people can get ordained online and start a church wherever. It does not mean because a person claims to be a minister or church that they are actually following Jesus.

There are abusers who maintain a twisted view of love because they were abused, or their concepts about love were tainted. Bullying, controlling, and lording over people can feel normal to them. It is not love, yet it fits their twisted perception of love. There are others who believe that men are supposed to dominate women, and that it was God's idea. They misunderstand who God is, misunderstand the Bible, misquote the Bible, and violate the greatest commandment of God, which is love. Domination and control are not love.

If we find a portion of the Bible that seems to violate love, then we probably do not understand the context or meaning. God is not double minded, nor the author of confusion. It is imperative to get to know the culture surrounding the Bible, the original language, and what certain terms meant to people in that culture. I have met people who believe they have the appropriate view of God and the Bible who have never read the entire Bible. They do not study the Bible. They do not look up the words in their original language. They do not study the context or culture. They will still grab a verse and beat another person to death with their understanding.

It is important to look at scripture as a whole; not just pick out passages and run with our ideas and interpretations. **There are parts of the Bible that merely tell a story of what happened in those places; it is not an encouragement to go do those things**. I will give you a few examples. David took Bathsheba as his own. David committed adultery and had Bathsheba's husband killed. This is not an invitation for other people to repeat what David did. There are people who completely miss the message of the Bible; they create abusive, oppressive systems or try to validate their mistreatment of others.

There were people in the United States who tried to use the Bible to validate their evil treatment of Africans in regard to enslaving African Americans. They attempted to use the Bible to legitimize slavery. The Bible does not tell you to hold people against their will, treat them like animals, hang them from trees, rape women, separate families, and abuse other human beings. The Bible states so plainly, "Do nothing from factional motives [through contentiousness, strife, selfishness, or for unworthy ends] or prompted by conceit and empty arrogance. Instead, in the true spirit of humility (lowliness of mind) let each regard the others as better than and superior to himself [thinking more highly of one another than you do of yourselves]," - Philippians 2:3 (AMP). Along with the scripture in Philippians, Jesus gave a warning to those seeking to exercise lordship over others. He stated that people in the world seek those things, yet the greatest in His family was a servant (Matthew 23:11).

Slavery of African Americans has ended in the United States, yet we are still dealing with the abuse of women and children. There is now a new monster to tackle. The new monster is human trafficking. Not all buyers of human slaves are non-professing Christians. There are men who claim to love Jesus buying slaves for sex, buying children for sex, forcing themselves on their wives, and behaving in ways that are anti-Christ. We hear on the news about hundreds of clergymen who were busted for molesting children and/or women.

What is even more disturbing than the abuse are the people who want to hide/defend abusers and pretend as though it is not happening. If you are hiding an abuser, then you are an accomplice. I have seen people rally behind a pedophile, rapist, or physical abuser in churches stating they are walking in love and forgiveness. I wish greatly people could understand that forgiveness and mercy are not forsaking wisdom and boundaries. God is just. God wants to heal the abused and the abuser. It does not mean we applaud the abuser; we set boundaries so more people are not abused in the future.

Abuse is evil and void of the love of God. There are people who twist the Bible to fit their selfish, or sensual agenda. Their agenda is void of the spirit of God. God does not regard humanity as commodities to be used, then discarded. God does not view people as objects to be used. There are people in the Bible who were sinful and did horrible things; this does not mean God approved of their actions.

Jesus did not arrive on the scene and say, "Here I am peasants, wash my feet." Jesus bowed low and washed their feet. Jesus served in sacrificial love. Jesus positioned Himself to love humanity, not oppress them. There is no one higher than God. When people position themselves to treat others with contempt, like sex objects, or without honor; they have completely missed God.

It is possible to have an idea or opinion about God, have head knowledge about the Bible, and completely miss the point. Jesus said He only did what He saw the Father doing, and only spoke what He heard the Father speaking. This does not mean that Jesus had no thoughts of His own or was a puppet. There are those who believe that God is domineering, controlling, and abusive. People will imitate the God they have envisioned in their minds. The lack of understanding who God is, and how God operates, can lead to major abuse. When a person does not understand that God is relational, God loves people, God does not use people, God is not selfish, God is not a bully, God allows people to choose, they come up with all kinds of ideas about how they should behave. Their behaviors can be anti-Jesus.

Jesus suffered abuse, because of sin, not because the Father is sick and twisted. If there had been no sin, Jesus would not have needed to go to the cross. The Father is not a sick, controlling abuser who enjoys the suffering of humanity. As stated previously, there was a purpose for the suffering of Jesus. There are people who are suffering for no reason at all. There are people suffering because of poor teaching on relationships, poor teaching on what submission means, poor teaching about what "head" means in relationships. There are people suffering because of misguided teachings on authority.

True godly submission is to be willing to yield to what honors God. It does not mean to obey or go along with what is sinful or ungodly. Submission also does not mean to blindly follow without contributing any input. There are people who do not understand submission, and therefore they are in oppressive, abusive situations. The Bible tells <u>ALL</u> believers to be willing to yield (submit) to one another out of reverence for Jesus (Ephesians 5:21). A good portion of what is preached orders wives to submit. Ephesians 5:21 is omitted.

There was a lady who shared a portion of her story in a training for an inner healing course. She was sexually abused from the time she was a child by her grandfather. The grandmother helped with the abuse because she wanted to submit to her husband. This is NOT godly submission. It is sin. Occasionally, what people call submission is encouragement to make a spouse an idol-place them above God.

We must stop teaching things partially or poorly. Why? One of the leading causes of death for a woman is abuse; not cancer, not heart disease, and not accidents. Abuse is killing women. Not only is abuse killing women, it is negatively impacting millions of children. It is an epidemic that **we cannot ignore**. Children who have been sexually or physically abused suffer greatly in life. We cannot keep telling women or children the following, "Whatever someone wants to do to you is okay. Submit to abusive leaders, submit to your abusive spouse, just love this person who is hurting you or your children. Your body does not belong to you, so if you just forgive, and give this person another chance, you will show them Jesus." This must stop and **we must hold abusers accountable**. I want to repeat the last sentence; there must be accountability for abusers.

We must teach what Jesus taught. **If a person does not love, they do not know God and do not belong in church leadership.** If a person is a pedophile, they should not be put over the children's ministry. If a husband or wife is abusing their spouse emotionally, physically or sexually, we need to stop telling them to try to save the other person. We must help the victim, and the abuser (if they want help). Let's stop chanting, "God hates divorce," so loudly and actually start to look at why people are abandoning covenant. Who wants to wake up to a person beating the snot out of them daily, yelling at them, or treating them and their children like garbage?

If we do not lift up a standard in communities of faith, we are missing out on part of the reason Jesus came. He came to set the captives FREE! He came to DELIVER the oppressed. He came to bind up the BROKEN. Right under our noses, people are dying at the hands of abusers. Under our noses, children are being violated. Under our noses, there is a gross misrepresentation of Jesus. Are we willing to be part of the solution? Are we willing to lift up a holy standard against abuse?

The major root of abuse is a lack of God's love and not knowing/abiding in God (1 John 4:8). He who does not love does not know God, for God is love. Along the same root, you will find insecurity.

Insecure people cannot love others because they do not love themselves. It is impossible to give away a love that one does not possess. If I ask a bankrupt person for money, they cannot give me anything. They may want to add value, but they are unable to do so. Insecurity leads people to seek to put others down to lift themselves up. Insecurity can lead to bullying and abuse. Every insecure person is not an abuser of others. Yet if you investigate abusers, you will find, at their core, issues with having a healthy love for self. As repeated over and over, we cannot love other people if we do not love ourselves.

Aside from ignorance of who God is and misunderstanding the Bible, insecurity is often the root of misusing the Bible to hurt people. Control is a fruit of insecurity. When people are insecure (fearful, lack healthy esteem, or have a fragile ego), they may seek to manipulate and control others. There are leaders who tell their people not to study or think for themselves. There are places where the pastor controls the congregation. There are those who try to force their spouse to submit to their wishes, and that is not love. There are those who are told submit, comply, or else. There are people who have been shunned if they raised a legitimate issue. There are those who may reject you if you do not agree with their interpretation of the Bible or verbally abuse those who disagree with them. Insecurity is not the path God paved for us.

I had a woman shun me because of a disagreement over the passages in Paul's letters regarding women and marriage. I spent years studying the Bible passages in their original language and studying the culture. She refused to listen and stopped speaking to me because I refused to agree with her. Love allows us to disagree with people without punishing them for differing opinions or differing interpretations. This woman repeated what she was taught and would not even consider her teaching was slightly off.

Jesus knew exactly who He was, and He loved perfectly. The person who has abused you, or is abusing you, does not truly know God or they are not abiding in God. These are not my words; these are the very words written on the pages of the Bible. The person abusing you may be dealing with their own issues, like the deep-rooted pain of being abused themselves. They might be struggling with their own demons (yes, there are spiritual forces at work with abuse), their pride (they think they are above love or above others), or they may be battling their own deep rooted insecurity. They may have strayed away from a personal relationship with Jesus or have stopped yielding to the heart of Jesus.

A person can believe in Jesus and still choose sin. John the apostle wrote, "I write unto you little children that you sin not, but if you do sin, we have an advocate with the Father, Jesus Christ the Righteous: and he is the propitiation for our sins: and not for ours only, but also for the sins of the whole world" (1 John 2:1-2). I have met people who believe that if you truly believe in God, you will never make a mistake or you cannot choose to sin. I wish this were true. However, we see in the New Testament words of correction directed at people who claimed to know Jesus. If you read Corinthians you will see Paul addressing issues in the church.

How do we deal with this in communities of faith? How do we deal with people who quote scripture, have been to seminary, have head knowledge, and yet they do not manifest the likeness of Jesus? I believe it is imperative that we look beyond talents, gifting, and credentials on paper. I believe we need to start examining the character of people, like the Bible instructs us. I am not encouraging becoming the sin police for people. I do believe we need to have proper discernment. Discernment is a spiritual gift that helps us to know the difference between what is right and what is almost right, between what is God and what is not of God. It helps us to determine where the boundaries need to be.

I also believe it is prudent that we teach people how to study the Bible, and how to know God for themselves. It is unwise to teach people to simply rely on their pastor or others to give them an understanding of who God is. I attempt to read through the entire Bible each year. We study entire books of the Bible in my fellowship. They are encouraged to ask questions, think for themselves, look things up, and know God for themselves.

I have encountered numerous abusive people, in communities of faith, who simply regurgitate what they have always been taught and emulate the behaviors they have seen. They prefer their opinions and traditions instead of the instructions God provided about love. They prefer to bully, control, humiliate, and hurt people rather than allow God to transform their hearts. I have spoken to a few people about their conduct over the years. They may have a grasp of what a Bible verse says; their demonstration is void of God love.

Tradition can hinder Jesus and the work of the Holy Spirit. There is such an obsession with male headship (meaning the husband is boss-the way it is often taught) in marriage and in communities of faith; there is complete lack of understanding of what those passages mean and God's heart. I have heard way too many sermons that completely miss God when teaching the role of the husband. The husband is not God, nor a god substitute. He is not Jesus, or his wife, the church. God gave a picture of Jesus and the church so that people could understand covenant, unconditional love, and mutual sacrifice. People have tried to duplicate the picture instead of gaining meaning from the picture.

God gave a picture of committed love, not lord and servant. Even Jesus stated, "I call you my friends." Even Jesus stated, "You will do even greater things." Even Jesus bowed low and served

25

sacrificially. Jesus, the King of all kings and Lord of all lords, positioned Himself to empower, to provide unselfish love, honor, protect, and to lift others up. True followers and believers in Jesus are seated in heavenly places with Him. True followers and believers are co-heirs with Jesus. We are not slaves, punching bags, or commodities of Jesus. God does not use us for His selfish gain. God is not selfish, vain, proud, or a controller.

There are people who believe that the pastor has ultimate authority and should be blindly trusted. This too is a misunderstanding of the Bible. I believe there needs to be a level of accountability in communities of faith and a ceasing of blindly trusting people who quote scripture or hold a position in a church. Please stop leaving children alone with pastors or people you don't know just because they are clergy. If a person states they are a Christian and can quote the Bible, it does not mean they are a safe person. There are children and youth who have been abused by youth pastors, youth leaders, and others by senior pastors. There are clergy who have misused the Bible to exert perverted authority. **God is the ultimate authority. When God calls a person to lead it is not for domination, control, mistreatment, or abuse.** Leadership, for God, is servanthood and sacrificial, unselfish love. We see these examples in the person of Jesus. He used His authority to help, bless, empower, develop other leaders, sacrificially love, and protect.

There are victims who have been abused by baby-sitters, family, or family of the friends of the child, who claim to be Christians. It's okay as a parent to say no to allowing your child to be alone with a person you have not thoroughly vetted. Please teach your children that just because a person quotes the Bible does not mean they have a right to force them to do things.

I recently went to Asia to serve with a ministry that focuses on rescuing women and children out of human trafficking. There was a rule that no one was allowed to be alone with a child. I told my team they were to minister in teams, not solo. It may seem like overkill, yet I believe it is far better to have too many boundaries to protect a child, than not enough. The ministry set up a buddy system. I knew a pastor who always had an administrator within hearing range during counseling sessions with the opposite gender or minors; that demonstrated wisdom. We cover boundaries in detail later.

Another area where abuse can occur is in pastoral counseling and mentoring. If a pastor or leader tries to force their will, it's a cause for concern. I have met with clients who have been told things by clergy that were gross violations of the Bible, yet they did not know the Bible well enough to know better. There have been clergy who encourage people to stay in dangerous or abusive situations because God hates divorce. They never mention God hates abuse. There are unfortunately people who use their position in the church as an open door to molest, oppress, and control. I think it is imperative to understand **clergy are not God replacements**. They are human. They can make mistakes and sin. It is wise to know God for ourselves and know the Bible too.

Check in on the clergy and find out how they are doing in their soul, and spirit. Just because they can preach the house down on Sunday does not mean they are okay or providing the truth. I have known women with dynamic husbands at church, but they were monsters at home. I have known people who put on a great show at church and were absolutely warped (perverted) in reality. No one checks on the condition of their spirit or soul. There are people who never question what they are taught. They do not study for themselves. They take another person's word; their lack of Biblical understanding can lead to abuse or control.

To recap this chapter, the Bible does not support a lifestyle of controlling, manipulating, or abusing people. Abuse is a fruit of not knowing God, not knowing God's love, and insecurity. Certainly, there are people who have slipped out of abiding in God and have for a moment or season, behaved in quite unloving ways. Hurting others and abuse is an indication of a disconnect from God. God is not abusive. The Bible is not a weapon to destroy people with or a tool of control. The Bible is supposed to provide a glimpse into the lives of people who encountered God, be a source of encouragement, parts are for guidance, and be a tool for relationship with God.

Abuse can also be the fruit of a person misunderstanding or intentionally exploiting the Bible. It is important for every person who claims to be a Christian to spend time getting to know God for themselves and not just take the Bible at face value. What would this passage have meant to the original audience? Are there other parts of scripture that seem to present another idea about this topic? Is this part of the Bible telling a story so we can learn that God will partner with broken people, or instruction on how to live? What did the original manuscript say? How does this part of scripture fit into the lattice of love? Where is Jesus in this passage?

What I would love for a person who was abused to know is that abuse is not God's plan. The abuser is not operating in God's love. We would love it if every person loved like Jesus. The reality is people can choose. They can choose to abide in God and love. They can choose to take parts of the Bible and twist it to fit their narrative. They can choose to follow their selfish desires and do what is evil. Jesus did not say His followers would be known by their church attendance, titles in the church, gender, professions of faith, or background. Jesus stated His followers would be known by their love.

If a person comes to you and tries to use the Bible to manipulate you, control you, or force you into doing things-this is a red flag. Jesus knocks on the door of peoples' hearts. Jesus does not push them open, nor hold people at gun point. Control and manipulation are fruits of insecurity.

Insecurity leads by control. Love leads by service, by being a servant, and having compassion. I met a lady at a church once who was quite manipulative and verbally abusive. She was able to get away with this behavior because we are called to just keep forgiving and not be offended. I confronted her. Why? She was sinning against me and others. She tried desperately to manipulate me into doing what she wanted. I pulled her aside and firmly but kindly told her, "This behavior is not okay. I will not be doing the things you asked of me." She tried to fight me on it, and I stood my ground and said no. No one had ever stood up to her by setting limitations. She tried to use scripture as a tool to guilt me into relationship. I said no. Forgiveness does not mean you will control my life. If a person is in danger, you don't tell them to remain in danger.

Once again, I highly encourage getting to know God and the Bible for oneself. I had a gentleman tell me once that we should not study for ourselves in case we get something wrong. I said, "How do you know if your pastor is right if you don't know the Bible for yourself?" There are so many things out there on the internet that are not Jesus, but people say it is. We must know for ourselves.

If you are struggling about the passages in the Bible about women and submission, I highly recommend the book, Why Not Women (see resources at the end of the book). It dissects Paul's letters and makes far more sense in the context of the rest of the Bible and God's heart, than the majority of what I have heard taught.

I want you to heal from spiritual abuse, misuse of the Bible for control or selfish gain. God is not a control freak. God does not appoint Hitler's over society. He allows choice.

Let's pray:

God, I want to know you, not just the things others have spoken about you. If there are things in the Bible I do not understand fully, please explain them to me. You hate abuse and when we are mistreated. Please remove any lies I believe about you because of my abuse. Give me your thoughts on who I am and what happened to me. I do not want to carry around brokenness. Heal me. Restore me. Help those who believe they are loving and it is abuse. Help them to see the error of their ways. Help those who are teaching things that lead to abuse. Teach them your ways. Please cleanse your church of abuse, mistreatment, and works of the flesh. We are called to love, and love does not abuse.

Questions:

1. What did you learn in this chapter?
2. What are some of the things you have been taught about leadership and submission? Have these ideas shifted after reading this chapter?

Chapter 3

When Sheep Bite or Devour (Getting Over the Wounding of Insecure, Immature, or Even False Disciples)

"Your love for one another will prove to the world that you are my disciples," Jesus (John 13:25).

I have heard numerous people quote the phrase, "Sheep bite." There are sheep who do more than bite, they devour. When I refer to sheep, I am talking about people who claim to love Jesus. Jesus is referred to as the Good Shepherd and those who love Him as sheep, in parts of the Bible. As stated in the previous chapter, expecting people who go to church and profess to know Jesus to always act like Jesus, is an unrealistic expectation. I would love to have Christians who act just like Jesus, love just like Jesus, and care just like Jesus. We are not living in a utopia. We are living in a fallen world that is inhabited by broken people.

Expectations can be a source of major hurt, when you are expecting those who claim to know Jesus to act like Jesus, to love like Jesus, to be there like Jesus, or even care like Jesus. **The truth is: expect Jesus to be Jesus** and understand that others are works in progress. There are mature Christians and those who are

immature. There are confident Christians, and some who are insecure. Some are being mended, and some are severely broken.
There are Christians who think they are following Jesus, yet they
are following a Jesus created in their own image. Jesus stated
plainly there are people who will claim to know Him and He will
respond He never knew them (see Matthew 7:21-23).

It is essential to understand that Christians are not the same in
their understanding of God, levels of submission to God, or behavior. I will state it over and over again; insecure people can
cause deep hurts in other people. An immature Christian may behave like a selfish toddler, or harm others simply out of ignorance.
Immature and insecure Christians may not reflect the heart or
character of Jesus in their actions. They may lack full awareness of
their identity in God and how to love like God. It is impossible to
love one's neighbor, if one does not love oneself. The way people
treat other people is often a reflection of how they feel about
themselves. A carnal Christian living out fleshly desires may behave just like a person who does not know God. There is nothing
in the works of the flesh that please God (Galatians 5:17). A person full of the love of God does not want to hurt other people,
control others, or abuse people.

Giving our hearts and trust to people just because they claim to
know Jesus is not wise. Trusting everyone who claims to love Jesus with our children is not using wisdom. Just because a person
sings Hallelujah, it does not mean they can be trusted with your
heart, your secrets, your time, or your children. The Bible is very
clear that everyone who claims to know Jesus is not really a follower of Jesus (see Matthew 7:21-22), that we should judge a tree
by the fruit it bears (Matthew 7:15-20), to guard our hearts
(Proverbs 4:23), to use discernment/wisdom (James 1:5, Philippians 1:9-10), and to test all things (try the spirit to see if it is of
God) (1 John 4:1-3).

Having the title of pastor or leader does not mean the person is of God. Church attendance does not mean the person is of God or connected to God. God is God. People claiming to be Christians are not God; therefore, expect imperfections. When perfection is expected of Christians, it leads to disillusionment. When people believe just because a person is clergy or a member of a church that they are perfect, it can lead to great disappointment. God partners with imperfect people and through relationship people grow in the character likeness of God.

I truly believe all people are capable of sinful behavior, biting others, backbiting, and committing hurtful, hateful actions. The problem arises when people have an expectation that Christians will never do these things. There is an expectation that those who claim to know God will act like God. It would be truly wonderful if every person who claimed to know God abided (remained in God) and manifested His likeness. The truth is that every human being has the capability to exert their own will.

God does not control people. I know there are people who shout, "God is in control." God is Sovereign, meaning nothing happens outside of God's knowledge. God does not control people like puppets. If God were a controller, Adam and Eve would have made appropriate choices. We would not have a sin problem if God controlled people.

Human beings can choose to sin which in turn creates problems all over the world. God is pure love. The Bible is very clear that God is love and those who do not love do not know God (1 John 4:8). Love fulfills the law because it does no harm to its neighbor (Romans 13:8-13). Therefore, **where we see a lack of God love, we see sin.**

God does not sin; humans sin. Sin is essentially rooted in selfishness and the desire to place our wants above what is right in the eyes of God. God is not the problem. Christianity (following Jesus) is not the problem. **The problem is sin.** Humans, even after a proclamation of loving God, can still choose to sin. God will not force anyone to refrain from sinning. Why? Forcing a person to do what we want them to do is control; that is witchcraft, not love. Love allows a person to choose. It does not mean that person is free from the consequences of their choices.

It is also imperative to note that a person does not become like Jesus in their mind, or emotions just by praying a prayer at a church. It is a journey. God invites people to enter into a relationship with Him. Before the Bible was written, God was present with relationship.

Part of the issue, I think, is that people stop at a prayer and do not mature spiritually to establish an intimate relationship with the Father. Therefore, they pray to invite God into their heart, and that's all that occurs. There is no mentoring, no discipleship (someone that comes alongside the person to help them), or teaching on how we actually establish a relationship with God. There arc people who do not know how to read the Bible, or how to talk to God, yet they are out there trying to represent God.

The issue is **we cannot represent a God we do not know**. Reading the Bible does not make us experts on God. In our everyday lives, we grow to know people by spending time with them, listening, going through life with them, and inviting them into our lives. When reading the Bible is construed as the relationship, people at times creates absurd ideas about God. Since there can be more head knowledge than actual experience, the person tries to continue their Christian walk according to what they know. There are people who repeat what they have been told versus what they have studied. I had a man debate me about the birthday of Jesus. I told him Jesus was not born in winter. He refused to believe that because he was always told December 25th was the birthday of Jesus.

When a person reads the Bible and, based on their understanding, sees God as one who loves to punish, they will punish others. The person who reads the Bible and sees God as sexist, will pursue and engage in sexist behaviors. We will imitate what we know. There are abusive people perpetrating the ideas about love and God they have been taught. They did not pursue knowing the heart of God. Not only do we imitate the God we know, we become like the gods we worship. It is possible to create a "god" in our own image that is not God at all.

I have seen an increase in biting Christians on the internet. We cannot tell from posts where a person stands with God. So, I will simply state the person professes to be a Christian online. The dialogue they start online can be combative, hostile, mean spirited, rude, and nasty. I have been called all kinds of names by professing "Christians." I have been called a heretic by people who do not even know me, their argument or judgement is based solely on their interpretation of the Bible. The person elevated their interpretation of the Bible above the command of Jesus to love. We can respectfully disagree with people. We can also ask questions: "Why do you believe this? Can you explain this?" We can take on an attitude of humility instead of pride. Pride is present when we are quarrelsome (Proverbs 13:10). The Bible says that "the servant of the Lord must not be quarrelsome, but should be gentle unto all men, able to teach, and be patient with difficult people" (2 Timothy 2:24).

What about outright abuse (spiritual, sexual, verbal, control/manipulation, or physical abuse)? These things go beyond just a disagreement or internet bullying.

There are people who are grossly insecure, and their insecurity leads to abuse. As stated previously, a person cannot love their neighbors if they do not love themselves. Putting you down, controlling you, manipulating you, and hurting you can be a means to deal with the internal conflict of self-hatred. There are abusers who claim to know Jesus, but they are not really following Jesus. Following Jesus leads to loving others (John 13:35).

Anyone can come into a church and pretend to know Jesus. They can quote scriptures, sing the songs, attend the meetings, and be just like the devil on the inside. Our understanding of what a follower of Jesus is must align with what Jesus said. Love, not church attendance would be the mark of His disciples. Love, not singing the loudest in church, or speaking in an unknown tongue would be the mark of His disciples. Love, in actions, not just in words, would be an indicator of who was His disciple.

I truly believe what hurts us the most is mistaking wolves in sheep's clothing for genuine sheep (those truly connected to Jesus). It is true that none of us are perfect; therefore, we may unintentionally hurt another person. A true follower of Jesus will repent (change their mind) and seek to turn from that behavior. A person who does not care who they hurt, or harm is not following Jesus. Jesus stated that if we abide in Him, then we will bear good fruit (see John 15:4-5). He did not say we would be abusive. Jesus is not abusive. That person who abused you was either 1. Not really a Christian 2. A Christian who chose to sin (violate God's standards). Again, God does not sin. God does not control, manipulate, nor abuse.

Spiritual abusers, those who use the Bible to try to control people, are often exhibiting the fruit of insecurity. Allowing people to think for themselves is dangerous and threatening to insecure people. It is a fear-based tactic. It also has a spiritual and demonic component. If you do not believe Christians can be influenced by evil spirits, well they can. I have far too many stories on the topic. The soul of a Christian can be oppressed, and any person can yield their will to what is ungodly.

Spiritual abuse can also be learned from other professing Christians. I have seen this with couples in marriage. Men are taught they are the head, which they interpret as boss (it does not mean that), and they abuse their wives. They ignore all the passages from Jesus about laying your life down, the greatest among you will be your servant, do not lord over others, love your neighbor as you love yourself, and seek to do no harm. They also forsake the example of Jesus, who being in the very nature of God, made Himself a servant, washed feet, and empowered His followers to do everything they saw Him doing. He did not limit them in any way. He did not seek to control nor boss them around. He walked with them and served. He loved sacrificially. He demonstrated what the Father is like for the world to see.

When the words of Jesus and the demonstrations of Jesus are placed below our understanding of the Bible, we have a problem. God, the highest of all authority, does not seek to control humanity. God does not seek to bully humanity. God visits the door of our hearts and asks to come inside to dwell with us. God does not bust down the door with weapons of mass destruction and force the Bible down our throats. Jesus did not say, "I am the Son of God, you slave. If you do anything displeasing, I am going to punch you in the face. Submit, weakling!" That is not the heart of Jesus.

Once again people will imitate the God they know. I also believe after reading the work of Brené Brown, that people are doing the best they can with the knowledge they have. I will give you an example from the Bible. Saul was a persecutor of Christians and a murderer, until he had an encounter with God. He thought he was doing the right thing, yet he was not. It took an encounter with the Living God to awaken Saul (*who became apostle Paul*) to his error. There are people, as twisted as it may sound, who think what they are doing is right. Before you jump out of your chair or throw the book down, think about this: we act on what we know. There are people who do harmful things because they have no example of healthy love. I jest not with you. Other people do harmful things because they are influenced by pure evil. Christianity is not the problem. I have had challenging experiences with hyper religious and insecure people in my lifetime. They have an idea about God and scripture. If you do not bend to what they deem is right, there are those who can turn into monsters on a witch hunt. I have also encountered clergy who want to control their congregations, so they don't want them to read the Bible for themselves, visit other churches, or have questions. Your pastor, and my pastor are not God. The same goes for a spouse. There are people who elevate a spouse to God status and use their role in marriage to dominate, control, harm, and abuse. Abuse is not godly behavior. Subjecting oneself to abuse is not godly either.

There are people who have been or are being physically abused by a spouse or parent. Please get help. Please call the domestic abuse hotline, 1-800-799-7233. You are not a punching bag. Abusers may claim they love the person, beat them up, then bring a gift to make up and quote scriptures about forgiveness. We can forgive people and not allow them to black our eyes. Yes, forgive. Also understand you were not created by God to be an abuse victim. You may connect with the National Domestic Violence hotline through the following link- https://www.thehotline.org/.

The other form of abuse that can be, and does show up, is sexual abuse. Any forcing or manipulation into sexual activity is not love. I know we live in a culture that promotes selfishness and lust. Society says that if you have a desire for someone, then you should be able to just have them. We are inundated with images that make people more like objects to be used than people to be loved. These attitudes can creep into marriage or dating. I have met both men and women manipulated into sexual activity by professing Christians. It's not just girls who are used for their bodies. Young boys, have been violated too. We were never created to be used or devoured.

In marriage, people can completely misunderstand Paul's advice to married couples about sex. I have heard those verses misquoted to mean any time your partner wants physical intimacy, you can force them into intimacy. Paul was addressing new coverts in the church of Corinth who wrongly believed once they gave their lives to Jesus, they needed to be abstinent. Paul told them because they were married, they were not sinning by being physically intimate. They were to come together in physical intimacy for the benefit of each other. I am referencing 1 Corinthians 7:3-4. It is possible to rape and sexually abuse a spouse. God created sex for love and intimacy, not force and control.

The Bible is clear on how we are to treat people. See the verses below.

Galatians 5:22-23 (AMP): But the fruit of the Spirit [the result of His presence within us] is love [unselfish concern for others], joy, [inner] peace, patience [not the ability to wait, but how we act while waiting], kindness, goodness, faithfulness, gentleness, self-control. Against such things there is no law.

Titus 3:9 (AMP): But avoid foolish and ill-informed and stupid controversies and genealogies and dissensions and quarrels about the Law, for they are unprofitable and useless.

Proverbs 29:22 (AMP): An angry man stirs up strife, and a hot-tempered and undisciplined man commits many transgressions.

Proverbs 22:24-26 (AMP): Do not even associate with a man given to angry outbursts; or go [along] with a hot-tempered man, or you will learn his [undisciplined] ways and get yourself trapped [in a situation from which it is hard to escape].

Romans 13:10 (AMP): Love does no wrong to a neighbor [it never hurts anyone]. Therefore [unselfish] love is the fulfillment of the Law.

1 Corinthians 13:4-7 (AMP): Love endures with patience and serenity, love is kind and thoughtful, and is not jealous or envious; love does not brag and is not proud or arrogant. It is not rude; it is not self-seeking, it is not provoked [nor overly sensitive and easily angered]; it does not take into account a wrong endured. It does not rejoice at injustice, but rejoices with the truth [when right and truth prevail]. Love bears all things [regardless of what comes], believes all things [looking for the best in each one], hopes all things [remaining steadfast during difficult times], endures all things [without weakening].

Yes, there are people claiming to be Christians and they are molesters, abusers, racist, sexist, controlling, manipulative, harmful, rude, and narcissistic. Just because they claim to be a Christian does not mean they are. As I proclaimed above, Jesus made it plain that "Many would cry out Lord, Lord," and He would reply, "Depart from me, I never knew you." (see Matthew 7:21-23). It would be quite easy for a person to just walk into a church and claim they are trustworthy. That person could be the world's most perverted or abusive person and be accepted. Jesus told us over and over to examine the character and behavior of a person's life.

One way we can take comfort is in knowing God will deal with false disciples. It does not negate the evil done, nor minimize the harm caused. I hope it leads us to cease trusting every person who claims to be a Christian. Do a background check before you allow an individual to work with children, make sure there are buddy systems in place, get to know people, look into a person's life before marrying them, investigate who a person is before you become best friends, and look for fruit (their behavior).

I know it may seem like overkill, yet I pray over every relationship and opportunity the following, "God show me who this person really is and remove anyone from my life who seeks my harm." God has been faithful to show me the hearts of people.

There are people who believe they are for you and they are not. Judas probably did not set out to betray Jesus, yet betrayal was in his heart. It does not mean we mistreat people if God reveals they are not for us. **It does mean we set proper boundaries.** The next chapter covers boundaries.

I want to note that we are not to stick our noses in the air even with people who are abusive. We don't know why they are doing the things they are doing. Several have been greatly abused as children. There are people who see their abusive behavior as normal. Pray for them. It does not mean you must be their best friend. It does mean there is most likely something inside that person that needs healed. It does not mean you need to be the person who helps them heal. I do recommend prayer.

I cannot tell you how many times it's come to light that the abuser has been abused. People who abuse others need help. If they want help, I think they can be helped. The key is does the person see the issue and want to be better? Once again, I do not believe it is the responsibility of the person being abused to save the one doing the abusing.

When the Bible talks about enduring suffering, it is not talking about allowing yourself to be molested, raped, consistently hurt, abused, or mistreated. People in the Bible were suffering for the sake of the Gospel, they were beaten and martyred for proclaiming Jesus. They were told not to retaliate evil for evil, but to overcome evil with good. Jesus suffered for the sake of the Gospel. It is not suffering for the sake of the Gospel to have no boundaries and just let people abuse us.

Prayer:

God, thank you that you are love. I submit all my memories from abuse from Christians. I was created by love, to be loved, then to love. I was not created to be abused nor to suffer mistreatment. I understand those that love you will suffer mistreatment from the world for following Jesus. I was not intended to be mistreated by other people of faith. We are called to love one another. I invite you to heal any and every part of me that has been mistreated or abused. It was not your idea. Reveal any lies I believe about you or myself from being abused. I release every person who has harmed me to you. I choose to forgive them (release them to you).

Questions:

1. What have you learned about sheep who bite or devour?
2. How does God feel about abuse?
3. How did you think about abuse from Christians before reading this chapter?

Chapter 4

Boundaries Are Vital to Thriving

"Daring to set boundaries is about having the courage to love ourselves, even when we risk disappointing others,"-Brené Brown.

Boundaries are necessary. God set a boundary in the Garden of Eden. He said to Adam, "but [only] from the tree of the knowledge (recognition) of good and evil you shall not eat, otherwise on the day that you eat from it, you shall most certainly [a]die [because of your disobedience] (Genesis 2:17 AMP)." God set a limit on what could be done in the Garden. Adam was given a directive and boundary. Adam ignored the boundary line and bad things followed. They did not drop dead from their violation, they introduced death on humanity. Humanity now suffers from mortality, sickness, pain, abuse, and so much more.

Boundaries protect what has value. There are people who could not stop or foresee their abuse. There are people who were abused because they did not set boundaries (limits, guidelines on treatment) with others. There are people who believe God will force another person to treat them with respect, honor, or dignity. There are people who ignore warning signs and it leads to future abuse. It is vital we understand that **we are responsible for setting boundaries and limits with people.** It is a lie that we are obligated to give everyone full access to our lives or we are mandated to friendship with everyone.

I have endured harsh things from Christians who believed after their abuse, I owed them relationship. We are to forgive (this means release the person to God and not seek revenge). We are not mandated to be best friends with everyone. Forgiveness is not the same as full restoration. God loves restoration, yet it is not always safe to be restored to everyone. Many domestic violence survivors who return to their situation do not make it out a second time. They are killed.

I met a lady in church and befriended her simply because we were in the same Bible study. Bible study is supposed to be a safe place. Over the course of our "friendship," she became more and more controlling and manipulative. She would purposefully test my limits and what I would tolerate. Example, I would tell her to forgo certain actions, because it made me uncomfortable, and she would do it anyway behind my back. Once she manipulated me into taking time off from work to go get her from a doctor's appointment. Supposedly, I was the only person who could come and get her. It was a huge inconvenience, yet I wanted to be a good friend and a good Christian. I was led by guilt and obligation. When I arrived at the clinic to get her, she was not there. She was at home. She called another friend to come and get her. When I called, I asked why she could not call me and let me know. She blew me off and stated she needed me to come sit with her because of her outpatient procedure. I unwisely went to her home to let her know, face to face, that it was not okay to have me use my vacation to come and retrieve her only for her to call another friend.

The only reason I volunteered was because she swore no one else could. Rather than apologize, she proceeded to tell me all her real friends were with her the night before to pray. I sat across from a woman who frequently attempted to manipulate me, publicly embarrass me, tried to control me through her interpretations of the Bible or what she thought I was doing, who volunteered to be my accountability person, because I needed one (which I said no to because it was a control scenario), and so much more.

My "friendship" with her wasn't a godly friendship; it was a nightmare. Any time she was confronted in love about her behavior, she either blew me off or started to cry uncontrollably for hours. She was always the victim. It was a horrible experience. Being in a relationship with her was like being slowly tortured. I was uncomfortable and unhappy. She was not pleasant and often unkind. She used her turn on the waterworks tears to manipulate and guilt people into relationship. If that did not work, she would quote scripture on how God wants us to be reconciled to one another.

I, in a moment of great desperation, changed my phone number and decided to not have anything to do with this woman. I was tired. I did not follow the biblical advice of confront, then go get others. Most of the people in my circle avoided her like the plague and did not want to confront her, knowing it would end in cycles of chaos. This woman went on to gossip and slander me to anyone who would listen. I had people contacting me at my job from the church about how awful I had treated this woman. One lady on staff at the church I was attending at the time, called me the b-word to my face in front of a table of other Christians. Though I was the person on the receiving end of pretty poor treatment, I was the villain because I did not want to endure it anymore. There are people who have called me names or a bad person because I refuse to be abused, manipulated, or allow people to waste my time on foolishness.

Let me tell you that **loving people does not mean becoming their doormat**. It does not mean becoming their punching bag. It does not mean you allow people to treat you like garbage and control your life. Part of love is learning to love ourselves the way God does. There were moments in my life when I would cry out to God and say, "Why have you allowed this person to treat me this way?" Or I would cry out, "God why don't you stop this person from hurting people?" Part of adulting is learning to set appropriate limitations, and establish healthy relating patterns with people. You and I can cry out for God to fix everything, or we can set limits with people.

I think there is a part of humanity that wants God to be their trunk monkey (commercial reference). In the trunk monkey commercial, there is this monkey in the trunk of the car or back of the truck. Any time the person gets into trouble, the trunk monkey gets out and handles the situation. You may liken the trunk monkey to a fixer. He just pops out any time there is an issue and makes people do what is right. Unfortunately, it does not work that way with God all the time. We have a role to play in forming boundaries with people. "No, you may not hit me." "No, I am not responsible for your feelings. If you are angry, that is your issue." "No, I did not make you do anything." "No, I am not allowing you to speak nasty and hateful things over my life." "If you refuse to talk to me with respect, I will disengage from this conversation and return when you can speak with kindness." "No, I am not allowing you to stay in my house with your abusive behavior." "No, I am not enabling you to continue to be abusive to me or my children." "No, I am not going along with your sin!"

Certainly, if you are in a situation that is life threatening, it is not always wise to tell the abuser you are not going to take it anymore. In cases of violence, getting help and getting out without them knowing may be the best option. There are people who have stood up to violent abusers and they backed down. There are others who have been retaliated against severely.

Occasionally in Christendom (the kingdom of Christianity) people are taught if they just love enough and act like Jesus, then the other person will see the error of their ways and stop abusing or mistreating them. Let me tell you that Jesus walked with the disciples and loved them well; Judas betrayed Jesus, and Peter denied Jesus three times. All of the disciples except John abandoned Jesus at His crucifixion. The women were there; the men He loved and discipled, except John, were gone. Jesus loved them perfectly, and they still chose not to love. We must stop teaching people that they are the savior.

There are people who won't even change for God. If people will not change for God, who is perfect, why do we teach people they will change for us? Yes, pray and walk in love. Part of love is wisdom. Wisdom is if a person is abusing you, seek help and set limitations on what is permissible. God cares about your safety and well-being.

It's God's will that none should perish. We still have people who perish. Why? They want to perish. It is not because God does not pursue with great love. You and I can do everything we know to do to love others, and they still remain the same. I have so many examples I could share with you about my attempts to love, love, love people who did not become more loving. They are still in sin and still hateful. Why? We can choose to accept or reject love. Why do we teach people that their human love can change others? It requires reception of love to be impacted by love.

God will also turn people over, who do not want to be loved or follow Him. Simply read Romans 1:27-29. God, the most powerful being in the Universe, does not force anyone to do right. Therefore, you and I need to use wisdom and set boundaries.

I heard a pastor say that women should not approach their husbands with boundaries, or correction; they needed to go to his head, God. The instruction was to pray about the situation or offense and not have a dialogue with him or correct him. Well this violates the passage of Matthew 18:15-16 (AMP) "If your brother sins, go and show him his fault in private; if he listens and pays attention to you, you have won back your brother. But if he does not listen, take along with you one or two others, so that every word may be confirmed by the testimony of two or three witnesses."

If your spouse is beating the crap out of you, you can pray all day, that may not stop them from beating you. Get help. If you cannot talk to them directly, seek help from the domestic violence hotline. I am very serious when I say, "Get help." If you are in a relationship with a person who is hurting you, understand that person has the capability to ignore God too. I hate when people do teachings on submission and headship, and they do not represent the heart of God. I could devote an entire book to the wrong teachings on these two terms. God does not want you abused. God does not set up systems of oppression.

I truly believe a chunk of the teachings, that tell women to just go along with whatever men say, is from hell. First, it leaves men with little to no accountability and an accomplice. If she must do what he says, then they both end up in sin. If she must do what he says, there is no one holding him accountable for his choices/actions. Studies have shown that men, frequently, have little to no close friendships outside their family, once they marry. So, his wife sees the majority of what is going on in the man's life.

We are not to be accomplices to sin, enable sin, or make God our trunk monkey (fixer). We set restrictions. We say no. We get support. We protect children. We do what is necessary so we can save a life. I also understand wives can be abusive as well. God did not design relationships for abuse. If you are being abused, please seek outside assistance.

If your church won't help you and screams, "God hates divorce, go home and submit, pray more, and just love the person," understand that I have seen people do those very things and end up in an extremely harmful place. There are people who die in those situations and that brings no glory to God. God hates when we are wronged. God won't force your spouse to change. God won't force any of us to change. There are cases where people have prayed their spouse out of abuse. I am not advocating for anyone to be a continual victim until their spouse stops abusing them. Set boundaries, set limits, and get help.

I wish there were more places where people, who are being abused or have been abused, could get help in the church. I know there are a few; I wish there were more. I wish there was more teaching on boundaries and abuse.

I spoke with a pastor I greatly respected about abuse in the church, and his reply was it was not his problem. If a person stated their spouse was abusing them, he would make them bring their spouse in and not just believe them. I told the person that expecting a person abusing their spouse to simply confess and never hit them again was unrealistic. At the root of abuse are issues that need godly intervention. I also explained that forcing an abuser to come to the initial counseling session, especially in violent scenarios, could bring more abuse. He did not have a grid for abuse or how abusers operate. Many are charming at church and monsters at home. I wish greatly there were more clergy who would stand up on Sunday and speak about abuse and how to set healthy boundaries.

Boundaries are limits we set in place to <u>protect</u> people. It's not about control. It's about protection. As stated in a previous chapter, I took a team to Asia, and we were working with women and children who were rescued from human trafficking or were still being trafficked. My team was given guidance on what was permitted. No one was to be alone with a child, ever! Men were not allowed to be alone with women (other than our team). They were not allowed to leave the mission compound alone at night. They were forbidden to go places in the city alone. Why? Even if we believe we would not behave improperly, that does not mean another person could not accuse us of improper conduct. Live a life that is above reproach. The guidelines were not given to control the team. The guidelines were given to protect the team. Also, if a teammate struggled with lust, they were never placed in a situation to be tempted above what they could bear. They had a buddy.

Boundaries protect what has value. If you go into an expensive jewelry shop and they have a million-dollar diamond, it is most likely locked up and you cannot touch it. There is also probably a mandatory guard for the diamond. You are more valuable to God that a million-dollar diamond.

If you are a minister, what boundaries are in place to protect the people God entrusted to you? What boundaries are in place to protect children? What boundaries are set to protect you? I have an assistant for inner healing sessions and documentation of sessions. I want to protect them, and I seek to protect myself. What boundaries are being taught at home?

God set us in families so we would have a first line of protection. Parents are to care for and protect their children. Unfortunately, there is abuse that occurs in certain families that creates a problem. The secondary problem is abuse in the world, and not teaching children proper limitations. My mother told me, I don't recall when, that parts of my body were off limits for adults. She explained if anyone did anything to those areas, I was to tell her, even if they told me not to, and I would not be in trouble. She also told me she would take care of me and not to be scared. Abusers often tell children not to tell because they will get in trouble. I knew if anyone tried to do anything to me, my parents would believe me. When I started dating, my mom told me certain things like, "Don't just accept a bunch of gifts from a guy (lavish things); some may think you owe them something for their gifts." "Always have enough money to get yourself home." "If something doesn't feel right, it is most likely not right." "Don't ever let a man get away with hitting you, if he does it once, he may do it again." "You do not owe a man your body." "How a man treats his mother and other women, is most likely how he will treat you."

On occasion people are mistreated by others because they lack adequate boundaries. I did not learn as much about boundaries with women/female friends. I soon learned that boundaries needed to apply to every area of my life. A lack of boundaries invites disrespect. People discern those who have little or no boundaries, and they respond to them with dishonor and disrespect. Emotional abusers will target people who are quick to forgive and those who do not set limits on their behavior. Many abusers test limits. They will do one thing, see if they can get away with it, then try again. The lady I told you about at the beginning of the chapter would test my limits, test what she could get away with doing. I would forgive her and try to love. She would wait awhile and then try again.

There are forms of abuse we cannot avoid. Example you come home, and your spouse is angry about dinner not being together and he slaps you around. You did not see it coming. What do you do now? What do you do when they say they are sorry and tell you that you must forgive because Jesus commands forgiveness? They promise to never do it again. I cannot tell anyone what to do. I can say that beating you up over dinner is abnormal. It is a major cause for concern. **How we respond to the first occurrence of abuse can determine whether it will happen again.** Physical abuse is not love. If a person hits you because you did not do what they wanted or disappointed them, that is not love. Love communicates and it's not with violence. There are times where people feel threatened and they lash out with violence, this is not a proper way to deal with issues. Blacking your eye is not communicating in a godly way.

It can be even more challenging, if the abuse is verbal or emotional and not physical. The person may say to you, "It's a misunderstanding. You are too sensitive." Put downs, public embarrassment, name calling, and hurling insults are not love. In those moments, I truly believe it's imperative to set limits and communicate. "Alice when you call me names, it is unkind. I do not like being called names." "Bruce, I do not like it when you put me down in front of others; it is dishonoring from my perspective." "Julie, when you give me the cold shoulder for three weeks because you are upset, I feel unloved and disrespected." "James, when you make fun of my weight, it is hurtful and unappreciated feedback." "Deon, I do not like the disrespectful communication. When you cool down, we can talk."

Communication is vital in relationships. The person may blow you off, or they may listen. I have dealt with people that no matter the spin you put on the information, they do not get what you are saying and continue to misunderstand. I have told quite a few people in my life that I did not appreciate their behavior. A few stated they were sorry, and things were mended. A few were offended and never spoke to me again. Either way it is a win because I set a boundary in love. When people love you, they will seek to honor your wishes.

We are not just called to love other people. We are called to love ourselves. Boundaries enable us to say to the other person, "I value who I am, therefore I can value you too." People who have no boundaries are often victims of abuse or mistreatment. They do not say no to what they do not want. Abusers normally violate boundaries and lack boundaries themselves.

As mentioned in previous chapters, people act out what they know. The man or woman who abuses their spouse may have witnessed abuse at home. That is their normal. I think it's vital to find out about a person's home life and what they interpret as love. It is prudent to investigate how they view gender roles too. There are men and women who are afraid and have control issues, therefore they seek to control other people.

It's not our job to change the other person. Our job is to set and reinforce limits. What we tolerate is what will continue. As soon as a person gets away with abuse, they learn that it is acceptable behavior for them. Maybe for that abusive person, forgiveness is offered, and a commitment to go to counseling. Maybe a spouse will say, "I never want to see a repeat of this behavior in our relationship. Something is obviously going on beneath the surface. In an effort to salvage this, let's set a time to speak to someone about your anger or (insert issue)." One, this moves the person towards understanding there is a problem. This wasn't just a mishap of, "I made a mistake and that's why I tried to throw you down a flight of stairs." Secondly, it gets the issue documented. Many times, domestic violence sufferers don't report it until it's been months, or years of abuse. Then the police or counselor says, "Well, why did you wait this long?" I am serious about people getting assistance; not to be perpetual victims of abuse.

Additional Notes on Boundaries (You are able to choose what works best for you. I am simply sharing what has been beneficial on my end, and from others I know):

Please talk to your children about appropriate and inappropriate touch. Let your child know to tell you of anything that makes them feel uncomfortable, even if the adult or other child abusers told your child not to tell you.

Please check with your church's childcare system and make sure they do background checks on staff, teachers, volunteers, and have a buddy system.

Please don't just leave your children with anyone, including clergy. Check people out. Do your homework, especially with teen babysitters. Check out the parents before letting your child go to another kid's home.

Please teach your children boundaries with other kids. "No, you may not touch me or talk to me that way." Bullying is happening and some parents don't realize children need to learn boundaries. Please talk to your kids so they feel they can tell you anything.

Set boundaries with people at church. Don't just trust a person because they are in church, leading a church, or in children's ministry. Don't assume that they are safe. At times, wicked people infiltrate communities of faith to harm people or children.

Set boundaries with your inner life. I do not share all of my business with everyone, nor give every professing Christian access to my life. I have certain people, who have proven themselves to be safe, that I share my world with them. Everyone else is on a need to know basis. Find out if a person is safe before you download all your inner world. There are people who are not mature enough to handle your story, especially if you are in the process of healing. There are people emotionally harmed simply because they did not share their heart with a safe person; they shared with a person who claimed to be a Christian. We have established that everyone who claims to know Jesus is not following Jesus.

I knew a lady from a community group, and I shared with her facts about some of the mistreatment I endured from other Christians. She was angry with me one day and said, "That's why people treat you like this…" and went on to berate me with things I had previously shared with her. **Pray for safe people**. I have safe friends outside Christendom; they are noble people. I do not trust someone just because they go to church, that they are godly. I have met evil people, dressed in street clothes, sitting in church.

Set boundaries with your time. "No, you may not call me any time of the day or night. If it's not a life or death emergency, then please call during these times."

I also learned I had to establish limits with serving. Occasionally when people know you want to serve and honor God, they will try to take advantage of you and make you a ministry slave. I learned to say no to what was too much or if I was being used. That person that always called to take up four or five hours of my day, talking about themselves, prompted me to stop answering the phone. I am not Jesus. He has unlimited time.

Set boundaries with who you choose to be a close friend. Just because in Christ we are brothers or sisters in the Lord, it does not mean we are to be best friends with everyone. I have endured unpleasant experiences in my life by befriending everyone at church. Some people you genuinely love them, but you do not make them a confidante or best friend.

Set boundaries with your body. Your spouses are not to force themselves on you sexually or abuse you physically. As previously stated, people can completely misinterpret Paul's instructions to the church of Corinth about the body of the spouse not belonging to them. He was addressing new converts who believed conversion to Christianity meant they were to be refrain from sex with their spouse. He was not saying that any time a spouse wants sex, no matter what is going on, you must do what they want. Sick and vomiting, too bad, here I come. That is not love. It is also possible to rape a spouse and it's not godly. Everything God does is rooted in love, not force.

Set boundaries with communication. If we allow people to talk to us like we are garbage, then they can believe it's okay. Enabling is not love. If a person calls me names for loving Jesus, they are ignored; it's suffering for the sake of Christ. If my "friend" calls me bad names, I tell them "No, that is not tolerated here."

Pay attention to warning signs early in the relationship: controlling behavior, needing to tell everyone what to do, unrepentant (hurts people and does not ever repent), more interested in looking godly than living a godly life, uses people, grossly selfish (thinks mainly about themselves), hateful, fits of rage/anger, mistreats other people, puts others down, mistreats their parents, excuses away sin, has no close friends (not even one), wishy washy behavior (Dr. Jekyll/Mr. Hyde), super secretive (no one can vouch for them), has two faces (public charmer/behind closed doors monster), overreacts to small things, super touchy, or has deep rooted insecurity. Every abuser has an issue with insecurity. Every person who struggles with insecurity does not become an abuser. Pay attention to how people feel about themselves. We can only give away the love we first possess. People who hate themselves cannot love you in healthy ways.

Even learning to guard our stories is a display of wisdom. I don't have the right to tell you how to navigate through your pain. I can provide examples on how to deal with pain. There are victims of abuse and mistreatment who are hurt because they do not provide boundaries for people regarding their story. They were hurt, raped, abused and now everyone has an opinion. I have never been raped, so I cannot speak to that person what they need to do. What I can do is offer love, compassion, and provide tools for healing if they are wanted.

The journey is between you and God. I have learned to tell people that I am not interested in their unsolicited advice about my story. It's not their story. Unless we live the story of another person, we cannot come with our basket of should's. I set boundaries with the "should" people.

I provided you guidance on things that have helped me, yet you get to choose how to walk out your healing. In the next few chapters I provide examples and tools. You can take what you need and leave what you don't.

Questions:

1. What boundaries do you have in your life?
2. Think of a time your boundaries were violated, what did you do?
3. What did you learn about boundaries in this chapter?

Abuse Red Flags Checklist

✓ **Controlling/Manipulative.** The person seeks to control you or others. Abusers may try to limit the person from having other relationships, even with their family. They may try to control the way a person behaves, what they wear, who their friends are, and where they go.

✓ **Verbal Put Downs.** Abusers may speak negatively to or about people then say "just kidding." It is a red flag if a person puts you down, talks down to you, constantly snaps at you, and speaks harshly to you. It's not love.

✓ **Violent Temper.** Many abusers will lash out and then come back with a gift and sob story. True repentance leads a person to change their mind about their behavior. The Bible warns against partnership with an angry person (see Proverbs 22:24).

✓ **Uses the Bible for Manipulation/Control.** The purpose of the Bible is not to control people. It's to provide insight into the work of God through imperfect people and provide guidance for spiritual purposes. It does not replace relationship with God. People had relationship with God BEFORE they had the Bible. Each person needs their own relationship and understanding of the Bible.

✓ **Has No Friends.** If the person has no friends at all, not even one, this can be an issue. The inability to maintain at least one relationship should be taken into consideration.

✓ **No One Can Vouch for the Person.** When you apply for a job, they ask for references. If you cannot find one person who can vouch for the person, this is a problem.

✓ **Unrepentant.** If you speak to the person about the issues you are having, and they do not take ownership of their part of the problem, this is an issue. Jesus told the disciples to be reconciled to the repentant, not to force relationship with the unrepentant (Luke 17:4). God actually requires repentance for reconciliation.

✓ **Won't Take No for An Answer/Pushy/Violates Boundaries.** No is a complete sentence. Do not touch me is a complete sentence. People who try to force themselves on you are not operating in love.

✓ **Super Spiritual in Talk Without the Fruit of Love.** There are people who are able to quote the bible all day, yet they lack any fruit of God love. Their walk and talk do not align at all.

✓ **Record of Abuse.** It is important to do background checks on pastors, leaders, children's ministers, and a person you would marry. Yes, I added marriage to the list. Marriage is a stronger commitment than a position at a church. There are people who fall in "love" and do no research on the person seeking to date or marry them. If they beat up their first spouse or are a registered pedophile, why would you want to marry that person?

✓ **Cruelty, Abuse of Animals, or Others.** If you watch a person demonstrate cruelty to someone else or an animal, understand that person is capable of doing that to you. Don't think if they are cruel to others they will not be cruel to you. If you see cruelty, it may not be you in the moment, that does not mean it won't be you in the future.

✓ **Holds Strong Negative Views About Certain People Groups**. I have never met a kind and loving racist or sexist. It is important to investigate how a person feels about people who are different from them or disagree with them.

✓ **Insecure and Self Loathing**. As stated before, a person who does not love themselves cannot love you. We can only love our others as we love ourselves. People who hate themselves cannot love you. We can only give away what we possess. It does not mean every insecure/self-loathing person is an abuser. It does mean most abusers are insecure/self-loathing.

✓ **Others Tell You to Run Away**. I have seen far too many people abused because they would not listen to wise counsel. They thought they knew what was best. If the people around you or people around that person tell you to run away, listen. I comprehend people are not always right. I also have seen people refuse to listen and end up in bad situations.

✓ **Comes on Too Strong, Too Much Too Soon, and Forced Intimacy**. Intimacy is built over time. If a person comes on super strong it could be insecurity, lack of understanding, or cultural differences. It could also be an attempt to gain intimacy without trust. Trust is built over time. When people do not take the time to actually get to know the other person, they can become entangled in the heart before they know the person is an abuser. With men, they may lavish a woman with gifts and complements to gain access. She may not take the time to check on his character. Women may offer a man their body thinking it is what he desires. Intimacy too soon is not the best route and may be a sign of insecurity.

✓ **Extreme Jealousy**. Jealousy can be a major issue. If you are dating a person and they are checking your phone, have angry outbursts over you being 5 minutes late, and constantly accuse you of cheating, it's an issue. It is especially an issue if you have not given them any reason to be jealous. It does not always mean the person will abuse you. It can be a catalyst for abuse.

✓ **Wants to Be Alone with Children/Minors.** There are people who love kids. I love kids. I do not try to get other people's children alone with me, with the exception of nieces and family for outings. I love when their parents come too. **If a stranger is <u>constantly</u> trying to be alone with your child or buddy up to your child, find out why.** There was a man from years ago I would always see playing with little girls from church by himself. It was not a one-time thing. He was a leader, so I did not pay much attention to him. Over time, I noticed it more and more. He was hyper focused on little girls. Years later (I left that church), I found out he was grooming underage girls for inappropriate sexual relationships. I am not stating every adult who wants to connect with kids is an abuser. I am stating there needs to be boundaries and investigation into the character of people who want to be your child's best friend. There needs to be investigation into those who ONLY want to connect with children/minors and not people their own age.

✓ **You Sense Something is Off.** I cannot tell you how many people have had a bad feeling and progressed anyway. If you feel something is off, stop, pray, and **<u>don't move ahead of peace.</u>**

✓ **Tries to Buy Your Affection.** I am not sure why gifts seem to be the route, yet in plenty cases of abuse the perpetrator used lavish gifts or grooming techniques to snare their victim.

✓ **Blames You for Their Bad Behavior.** You made them angry. You are the problem. It's always your fault. Blame shifting can be an abuser's best friend.

✓ **Pastors Frequently Counseling/Ministering to Opposite Gender/Children Behind Closed Doors Alone.** This has gotten a few leaders in trouble. It does not mean abuse is occurring; it is an area to exercise caution. There was a leader all over the news for an inappropriate sexual relationship with a woman he was counseling. She had a sex addiction, and he was "ministering" to her behind closed doors, one on one sessions. Shun the mere appearance of evil. In children's ministry or work with minors, have another person present. In opposite gender meetings, do what you can to have transparency. My old pastor had an office with glass walls and an admin would sit outside meetings. There was no opportunity for physical or sexual abuse. I do not do sessions with minors alone. Their parent must be present. I have a trained assistant for inner healing sessions and they are present for all in person sessions. Sessions are also audio recorded with the client's permission. If a leader constantly has closed door "meetings" with minors or those of the opposite gender, this may be a set up for abuse. There have been cases of same sex assault as well. **If you are a leader, think about boundaries to protect yourself from false accusations or a person stating you did something inappropriate.**

This list is not exhaustive. It includes things I have noticed over the years with people and in study on abuse. Abusers seem to love control, hurting people, and satisfying their selfish desires at the expense of others. If we can pay attention to warning signs, it can save us so much pain and hurt. The lady I wrote to you about earlier in this chapter had red flags I ignored at first. She did not have very many friends, and the ones she had spoke badly about her at times. She was controlling and pushy. She put me down publicly and was unrepentant. I wanted to be a "good" Christian and love her. I failed to see, at the time, that God expected me to love myself as well. If I had paid attention to the initial issues, it would have saved me years of madness. Are you paying attention to the red flags?

Chapter 5

Is Forgiveness Enough?
(Healing is More Than
Forgiveness)

"We must develop and maintain the capacity to
forgive. He who is devoid of the power to forgive is
devoid of the power to love. There is some good in
the worst of us and some evil in the best of us.
When we discover this, we are less prone to hate
our enemies,"
-Martin Luther King, Jr.

Healing is more than forgiveness. I wish I could tell you that the moment you forgave the person who harmed you, the heavens would open, and you would feel like it never happened. Unfortunately, it does not work that way. We are triune beings; body, soul, and spirit. When we are abused or mistreated, all three register what has happened. That bruise on your face may heal, but what do we do about the bruise on your soul? What do you do with the memories that recur over and over, and the waves of negative emotions? What do you do with the pain that creeps up stealthily at midnight leaving you like the victim of an awful horror flick? What do you do when the sight of that person, or the smell of their cologne, triggers nausea and pain? What do you do when going back to that church, or that office, makes your body react with the same traumatic sensation you experienced when the abuse initially happened?

I hear people in Christendom shout forgive, yet not many Christians actually deal with the aftermath. You have forgiven and released that person to Jesus. It is expected that you are now best friends, or your marriage is perfect, because forgiveness is the magic pill. I will tell you the pain does not cease at the moment of forgiveness. It does not stop the moment you decide to say, "Okay God, what this person did was sinful and awful. I release them to you." Your soul remembers how it felt when the abuse or mistreatment occurred. Your body remembers how it felt to be struck or violated. Your body and your soul see a perpetrator every time they look at the person who harmed them. You can pretend to have warm fuzzy feelings, or you can face reality.

If I take a china plate and throw it on the ground and smash it into thousands of pieces, it is broken. If I take a can of gasoline and matches and burn your house to the ground, you have ashes. If I take my car and run you over fifty times, you will be in a body cast or dead. Asking you to forgive me does not put the plate back together, rebuild you a new house, get you out of the body cast, or raise you from the dead. The moment I say I am sorry and ask you to forgive me does not magically fix all the problems. Oh, but what about all the Christian movies that have the happily ever after; the husband decides to stop cheating and abusing the spouse simply because of forgiveness. It's magical! I wish they would show the families that walked through painful counseling and the laborious task of rebuilding trust.

Forgiveness only opens the door for rebuilding and restoration. God is the one, with our participation, who puts us back together again. Forgiveness, from my experience with life, and working with abused people, does not heal the pain caused by the infraction. It opens the door to clean out the wound, so an infection of bitterness, resentment, pain, and revenge do not take up residence in your soul. When we do not forgive, the pain the person inflicted upon us continues to hurt, to fester, and continues to cause ongoing pain. Resentment and bitterness are horrible bedfellows. Malachy McCourt once said, "Resentment is like taking poison and waiting for the other person to die" (Anderson, 2015, para. 1).

Bitterness hurts the person who refuses to forgive. When we refuse to surrender the person, who hurt us to God, we are twice as wounded. We are wounded by the person who hurt us and wounded by refusing to release the hurt. Letting go is not approving of the other person's behavior. Letting go is not refusing to get help or neglecting to punish perpetrators. Yes, we love even our enemies. We also **set boundaries and limits on reckless people**. We do not leave children alone with child predators. We do not keep a person in a position of senior leadership, who is beating their spouse at home. Forgiving is not giving a person a free pass to keep abusing people. God is not insane. He is not saying, "I know that pastor molested you, please be alone with him again and hope he will not do it again."

When I have sessions with people for deep inner healing and soul care, there can be push back in the area of forgiveness. There is an inner fear that forgiving is letting the perpetrator off the hook. I have seen those memes on social media where people are angry at God and at Christianity because they believe it's a free pass religion. It's not a free pass religion. When a person genuinely repents (which is more than throwing a sloppy, "I'm sorry" on an issue), God takes care of the eternal consequences for sin. It does not take care of all of the earthly consequences for sin. If you rob a bank, God can and will forgive you, but that does not mean you will walk freely on earth. Forgiveness is **not** a free pass in the sense that we can do whatever we want and never suffer any consequences for our actions. It is not a free pass where all the pieces of our lives magically revert back to the way they were, as soon as we apologize. If trust has been broken, it can take time for trust to be restored.

I am troubled by people who have never been abused, or ever worked with abuse victims, who are quick to tell people, "Just forgive," like it's no big deal. They do not have the painful replay, the memories, or the experiences of wounded individuals. One of the things I love about God is this: He is not haphazard in His approach with people. When I have sessions with people, and they unveil their horrific experiences, Jesus is not yelling at them across the way saying, "Forgive!! If you just forgive, I will help you." I notice that Jesus is ultimately concerned about the person and the connection with their heart. There are times I have noticed people treating other people like projects, instead of people. We complete projects; we have tasks associated with projects. The project goal with abuse victims can be to get them to forgive and immediately forget what happened to them. God longs to listen to and heal the person. Love seeks to heal.

The goal of Jesus is relationship with humanity. When Mary and Martha were upset about the death of Lazarus, Jesus responded to each of them based on their relationship with Him. We see two different women approached in two different ways. When we are dealing with our own pain, or the pain of others, I believe it is vital to understand that Jesus loves people. Jesus does not treat us like projects to fix; we are people He loves.

God is the master carpenter who delves into the rubble and ashes to rebuild, repair, and make things better than before. You may be thinking, "How can I say such a thing? How on earth could your story be better?" I simply follow what I have seen in my own life and the words spoken about Jesus. I will give you more insight in the Victim to Victor chapter.

We see in Isaiah 61 there is hope in Jesus. He comes to bring good news to the humble and afflicted, bind up the broken-hearted, proclaim release to the captives, freedom to prisoners, to comfort those who mourn, give joy instead of mourning, praise instead of a disheartened spirit, beauty for ashes, a double portion instead of shame, and reconstruction of the ruins.

Exaltation of the Afflicted (Isaiah 61:1-7 AMP)

"The Spirit of the Lord God is upon me, because the Lord has anointed and commissioned me to bring good news to the humble and afflicted; He has sent me to bind up [the wounds of] the brokenhearted, to proclaim release [from confinement and con-demnation] to the [physical and spiritual] captives and freedom to prisoners, to proclaim the favorable year of the Lord, [And the day of vengeance and retribution of our God, to comfort all who mourn.

To grant to those who mourn in Zion the following: To give them a turban instead of dust [on their heads, a sign of mourning], the oil of joy instead of mourning, the garment [expressive] of praise instead of a disheartened spirit. So, they will be called the trees of righteousness [strong and magnificent, distinguished for integrity, justice, and right standing with God], the planting of the Lord, that He may be glorified.

Then they will rebuild the ancient ruins, they will raise up and restore the former desolations; and they will renew the ru-ined cities, the desolations (deserted settlements) of many genera-tions. Strangers will stand and feed your flocks, and foreigners will be your farmers and your vinedressers.

But you shall be called the priests of the Lord; people will speak of you as the ministers of our God. You will eat the wealth of nations, and you will boast of their riches.

Instead of your [former] shame you will have a double portion; and instead of humiliation your people will shout for joy over their portion.Therefore, in their land they will possess double [what they had forfeited]; everlasting joy will be theirs."

Forgiveness helps to clean out the wounds so we can be healed. We don't want bitterness and hopelessness to take root in our souls. Enough damage has already been done by the perpetrator. We don't want to keep being victimized. I see clients who have been raped and severely injured. I want them to be free, not in perpetual bondage. Unforgiveness can become like an infection in a wound, it prevents the wound from healing properly. We must clear out the infection so the wound can heal. There is a difference between saying, "Forgiveness causes instant healing," and "Forgiveness facilitates wholeness." Whether there is an infection in a wound or not, there is a wound present. Even when a person forgives, there is a healing process.

Process can be such a swear word to people. We live in such a fast food society that says, "I asked for this, you have 60 seconds to make this happen." I see this in inner healing sessions with a few clients. They come in with 30 or more years of baggage and bondage. There are a few who expect their entire lives to be fixed in one session. One, I am not a fixer. I facilitate an environment for people to navigate through their pain. Two, part of their healing involves their participation and cooperation. They leave with homework and have things to do before each session. I survey people after the session ends, and the ones who do the homework or their part, often have the best results.

I wish one prayer of forgiveness took away years of pain, yet that has not been my experience. My experience has been that forgiveness is an act that may be repeated over and over. It is a decision of the will to leave the final judgement to God. It can involve surrendering a person over and over again. "Dear God, here is this person who hurt me again. When I think of them my heart still feels (insert what is happening in your heart). I surrender this person and painful situations to you. Free my heart of attachment to this person who is unhealthy."

Ask God to reveal anyone you still need to forgive. If there is a name or list of names that comes to mind, go through the prayer on the previous paragraph. Release the person to God. Release what they did to hurt you to God. God can handle all the negative emotions, pain, and trauma. More than anyone else, God can handle it. Releasing a person to God does not mean they are not guilty. You are not forgiving an innocent person. **You are releasing a guilty person to God for Him to deal with appropriately.** Trusting God with a person who has been abusive is not always easy. I will on occasion ask God to show a person the spiritual age of the person who hurt them, or reveal truth about their abuser. Quite a few have seen their abuser as a wounded or confused child.

Ask God to reveal any lies the abuse has caused you to believe. Maybe one of the lies is, "This is my fault. I am so stupid for trusting this person." I often ask people in sessions to ask God to show them where He was when they were being mistreated and abused. There is comfort in having the knowledge that no person is alone during a traumatic event. Though God does not prevent all trauma, God does not leave the room. One lady told me she had an impression of Jesus with her in the room, crying. One lady told me she had an impression of Jesus blocking part of the harm the person intended. God allows people to choose, and I know it's a challenging concept to grasp when we are on the receiving end of the abuse or mistreatment.

Maybe the person you need to forgive is the person who is looking back at you in the mirror every day. Maybe the person you trusted was the wrong person. You believed the best, but you received the worst. Maybe you trusted a leader with your child, or another person with your child, and they were a predator. As humans, we cannot prevent all harm, though we would love to do so. We can be blind sighted by people.

Maybe you are at the point where hearing the person's name or saying the person's name triggers pain. If that is the case, take heart. I know it's easier said than done. Maybe hearing the person's name triggers memories that are so painful you can barely breathe. Maybe hearing their name causes deep pain and trauma. Maybe seeing their face is similar to reliving the horror again. If you are in that place, the next chapter on soul healing is for you. There are times when the trauma is so severe, a person needs soul healing prior to being able to start the process of forgiveness.

Imagine having a back pack, and every time a person hurts you they add a heavy stone to your back pack. You are trying to climb a mountain, yet the stones are heavy. The moment they hurt you, there was pain inflicted. The heavy stone is also breaking your back. Jesus comes along to walk with you. He asks, "Can I take those heavy stones from you?" You have a choice. I have a choice. Keep the stones, or hand them over. Handing over the stones is not saying they are not heavy. It is not saying the person who caused the hurt is right. It is getting a load off your back.

I have encountered people who were unable to forgive until we invited God into the painful memory. The memory had to be addressed before they could release the person. Are you stuck? Are you replaying anger and resentment towards a person or numerous people? God longs to free every person from the pain of abuse. Being abused is the first mark of pain, leaving the wounds unhealed and refusing to release the person who harmed you is another level of pain.

Let's get rid of heavy stones!

Ask God who is a heavy stone on your back. You are still carrying negative emotions towards that person.

Prayer:

God, thank you that you wish to heal all the pain caused by (insert the person's name). I do not want to carry these heavy stones any longer. I want to be free. Please come into all the painful memories caused by (insert the person's name). Clean out all the pain there. Heal all the negative emotions and pain caused. I release them and this situation to you. I give (insert person's name) to you. I no longer want to carry any unforgiveness, bitterness, resentment, anger, or hatred towards them. I choose as an act of my will to surrender this person to you. I am not forgiving an innocent person. I am forgiving a guilty person. I want to be free; I cannot be free while holding onto them. I release them from my soul. Help them please not to hurt others and to know your love. Lighten my load. Thank you for taking my pain and hurt. In Jesus name. Amen.

Chapter 6

Deep Inner Healing
(How to Get the Junk Out of the Soul-So the Abuse Does Not Kill You)

"Beloved, I pray that in every way you may succeed *and* prosper and be in good health [physically], just as [I know] your soul prospers [spiritually]," (3 John 2:2 AMP).

As I stated before, we are tripartite consisting of a body, soul, and a spirit. When abuse and mistreatment occur, it's contrary to how we are supposed to be treated. We were created by love, to be loved, then to love. Abuse is not love. Mistreatment is not love. Since we were created for love, mistreatment and abuse can cause wounding to the body and soul. The wounding to the soul (mind, will, and emotions) can be mild or severe. There are people who are able to brush off mistreatment easier than others. There are those who have a history of mistreatment and abuse; they may have a greater difficulty recovering.

One of the illustrations I use in soul healing classes with people is imagine your soul as a piece of fruit. If you take that fruit and throw it on the ground and trample it, it will bruise or break open.

If we do not deal with the bruised (wounded) parts, they do not supernaturally disappear. The bruised and wounded parts do not instantly heal. If you take a piece of fruit that has been damaged and sit it out, the broken parts will begin to rot first. Bugs and rodents go after the rotting parts. The bruised and wounded parts are also vulnerable to future injury.

I have encountered people who have been carrying buried trauma since childhood. It was never dealt with so it never healed; it simply sat there. Since they carried unhealed wounds of abuse, many attracted more abuse. Woundedness can attract more wounds. Abusers can sniff out those who have been previously abused. It is essential that things that have hurt and wounded us are dealt with and not swept under the rug.

Negative emotions that we bury do not die, they lay there, and many times resurface in our worldview and responses to people. The person who has been abused may struggle to trust any person again, they may run from intimacy (connection with others on a healthy deep level), may have unhealthy defense mechanisms, or may develop an attraction to people who have the same abusive tendencies. It is not uncommon for me to see people in sessions who were abused as children and then went on to date a person who was abusive or attract friends who were abusive.

I had a lady who was abused as a very young child. She was singled out by abusers over and over. It was as if she had a target on her that said, "Please abuse me." It was not her fault. Her initial abuse was never healed and never dealt with, so the abusive pattern repeated itself over and over in her life. It sent out a signal "Abuse me again!"

We want to break cycles of abuse and patterns of abuse. It's most likely not your fault you were abused. Choosing to live with unhealed hurt is a choice.

I have heard people misquote the verse that says, "We press onward and forget those things which are behind." They use this to say that we should just forget about what happened, pretend the abuse is not an issue. Well buried pain does not just heal. Think about that bruised fruit, does that bruised or broken off piece return to healthy on its own? No, it does not. Does that plate smashed on the ground glue itself back together? No, it does not. We have people walking around who look whole on the outside and inside they are still broken. There are people I have encountered with distinct broken parts that are a different age. They suffer from what is called dissociation. They have been traumatized so greatly a part of their personality fractured and holds the painful memories and experiences. These parts, from my study and experiences with people, do not go away because you ignore them.

Certainly, minor infractions, like someone accidentally hurting your feelings, can be easily recovered from and potentially easily forgotten. I am not talking about minor things that happened to people as adults. I am speaking of severe abuse, and things that hurt so deeply it wounded the soul. There are wounds that can occur early in childhood, when the coping mechanisms are low, that still need to be healed as adults.

I had a woman in an inner healing session who struggled her entire life with closeness and intimacy with other people. Her failure to bond intimately was the result of her being placed in an incubator as an infant. She perceived as an infant, that she was abandoned by her parents. How could a person recall back to that age? We are a body, soul, and spirit. A baby cannot talk to you, but it does have a soul that is logging memories. The inability to talk, does not mean the baby does not have feelings, or that they are completely oblivious to what is happening around them. They can feel pain, loss, fear, and other emotions.

There are situations where the abuse has been severe. In cases like this, people can repress the memories and be unaware that there is deep rooted resentment or pain in the soul. If you are struggling and witnessing recurring patterns of abuse or mistreatment, there may be a problem with a soul wound, or numerous soul wounds, that need healing. I encourage seeking help with someone trained to help you.

If you are struggling with connecting with people or God, find yourself overreacting to things that others find small, have frequent nightmares, suffer from self-loathing, seem to attract the same negative circumstances or types of negative people, there may be a wound or series of wounds on the soul. Addictions can also be a cry for comfort and an outward manifestation of a soul wound.

We established in the last chapter how forgiving does not put the smashed plate back together. Ignoring the bruised part does not remove the damaged parts. I know there are people who believe you can find wholeness through one prayer. They argue against deep inner healing or any other methods. My goal is not to argue or try to convince anyone to change their mind. I simply share from my experiences with people and training in this area.

God can do anything, one touch and bam that person can be completely made new. I have met people who have been through regular counseling and prayer without any change. They are still stuck, still hurting, with plenty blaming themselves. They believe that if they had enough faith, then they would already be healed of their emotional pain and be whole. I have encountered those who have prayed, read the Bible, done all the church things, have forgiven others, and they are still carrying the pain of abuse.

How do we go about healing? I want to share with you just a few things I learned from Dr. Kraft and Dr. Bitcon. First, we invite God into the memory and the incident. Instead of pretending the event did not happen, we invite God into the memory. Second, we recognize the negative emotions that surface because of the abuse or mistreatment. Third, we deal with the negative emotions. I also ask people to speak out verbally, anything they grew to believe because of the abuse and mistreatment. What is God's truth about the situation and the abused person? Truth is a powerful tool. It's amazing the things we can grow to believe because of abuse.

Inviting God into the memory is a tool to recalibrate the situation. Instead of the person enduring the situation alone, they can begin to see that they are never alone. Many people have shifts in their opinions of themselves after their healing session, and about what happened to them.

Recognizing the negative emotions that surfaced during the incident is equally as powerful. Examples of negative emotions may be fear, shame, pain, hatred, or insecurity. Navigating through these negative emotions with God is a liberating experience. Instead of pretending they do not exist, or burying them, they are handled. I love what Dr. Kraft states about unhealed negative emotions, "They are like garbage that the rats come to feast upon." Soul wounds that are not healed attract the wrong things, the wrong people, and even unwanted spiritual intruders. I had a lady who was gang raped and after that experience, she would have nightmares of being raped. She was plagued by nightmares and heard voices taunting her. The voices and nightmares stopped after her soul healing session. We do not want to leave the garbage in the soul.

I ask clients for the lies they believe because of abuse or mistreatment because when we believe the lie, we empower the liar (the devil). Abuse attacks identity. We were created for love, not abuse. When people abuse or mistreat us, especially clergy or professing Christians, it can create a fracture in our beliefs about ourselves and God. A common lie I have heard is, "God does not love me. If God loved me, He would not have allowed this abuse." Another common lie is, "I am worthless because I was abused. No one will ever want me." A frequent lie is, "I am unlovable." The list of lies can be excessive. What we believe, we empower. There is power in our thoughts and what we believe. The person who has been abused, who begins to believe the lies that resulted from their experiences, can be re-injured over and over by a lie.

It is necessary to examine beliefs about the abuse and mistreatment and impart truth. It is not the truth that ultimately sets a person free, it's **believing the truth that sets people free.**

Imagine walking around daily believing that you deserve abuse, God does not love you, or your abuse does not impact God. There are people walking around bleeding on the inside. They are singing songs on Sunday and depressed the rest of the week. We wonder why addiction is so high. As stated before, addiction can be a huge cry for comfort. There is pain, and there is a desire to mask the hurt, numb the hurt, and avoid the hurt. Some are cutters, some overeaters, some drinkers, some addicted to social media, some serial relationship people, and some cannot function without an illegal substance.

Part of what I do is serve the homeless on the streets of my city. Often, the addicts I see with tracks in their arms also have deep rooted soul wounds. One heroin addict I met on the streets was abused as a child. That wound was never healed. So, she medicated herself to avoid the memories and the pain.

I had another person we tried to help for years who was chronically abused. The person was a Christian, but they were not functional. They battled anorexia, bulimia, cutting, destructive behaviors, and much more. They did the Christian things we tell people to do such as praying and forgiving, and the person was still in agony.

The buried pain can scream out for help and healing. There may be a little girl, or little boy, on the inside crying out for healing and restoration. Maybe you have heard the nagging voices that cried out for help, that cried out with negative emotions, and did not find comfort in just forgiving. Maybe you have tried forgiving, yet every time you think about what happened to you there is tremendous pain. Dealing with the negative emotions attached to the wounding is not weakness; it is wisdom.

I had another lady who was picked up by a stranger on the way to school and he raped her. She heard this nagging voice her entire life, "It was your fault." This one incident followed her for the duration of her life. In two sessions, we were able to address the 12-year-old part of her; it was still holding trauma, abuse, and a host of negative emotions. She reported back after her sessions that they were life changing for her. She no longer heard the voice. She felt for the first-time, confidence and closeness to God. There were numerous lies about God and herself that she had believed because of the abuse.

One chapter simply will not suffice to cover everything about soul healing. I wanted to introduce the topic to you because I am passionate about freedom for people. I am equally interested in people finding hope. I care about those who have been displaced and cast aside, when the methods of merely praying and reading your Bible have not worked for them.

I have encountered people who love God, and their soul is shattered. They have done everything in their power to be made whole, yet they are still in bondage. Jesus paid for freedom, not bondage.

Have you been greatly wounded by a leader or person in the church or abused by them? God does not desire for you to carry that with you for your entire life. **Yes, they hurt you. The goal is not to carry that pain forever. It can be removed.** No matter how deep the wounds go, or how long the abuse was endured, there is healing available.

What painful memories are being suppressed in your subconscious or conscious mind? God knows. What situations seem to be too unbearable? One of the things I have clients speak out at the beginning of every session is, "God whatever you want to heal in my heart and soul today, I want it to be healed." I do not go on a scavenger hunt of hurt with people. I invite God to bring forward any memories that need to be healed.

The simplest activity I can give you is to follow the cliff notes I gave you earlier in this chapter and in the activation section below. These are simple steps and I am not guaranteeing total freedom or effectiveness for every person.

There are wounds that are easily dealt with by ourselves. There are other wounds that are so deep or hidden they may require additional help. God is the primary, since God knows everything and operates in perfection. There is no shame in seeking help. Having a deep inner healing session with another person can be one of the best ways to process the hurt and pain. I have, at times, recommended to people counseling to assess their mental health and habits.

Simple on your own soul healing activation:

Set aside time to do this activity; do not rush through the steps. You may want to grab a pen and paper for documentation.

1. **Ask God to reveal any unhealed parts of the soul**. A memory may come to mind or a person who harmed you (wait and listen).

2. **Invite God into the memory.** Ask God to show you or tell you where He was during the event. Ask God for His truth regarding what happened (wait and listen).

3. **Identify the negative emotions** that surface from the event. Examples may include shame, embarrassment, fear, or anger. You can pray out, "I break the negative attachment and hold (insert negative emotion) has over my life and command everything that came to reinforce (insert negative emotion) to leave me and go to Jesus. God replace (insert negative emotion) with your love." The greatest healing often occurs in step 2. Step 3 is clearing out the negative emotions attached to the wounds. It's okay to take time and address what you are feeling with God. God is not put off by your anger, resentment, (fill in the negative emotions). He can tolerate the tears, anger, and deep sorrow.

4. **Ask God to reveal any lies you believe because of the abuse and mistreatment.** Renounce, and come out of agreement with those lies. You can make your list of lies and then go through them: "I come out of agreement with the lie that the abuse was my fault, I renounce that lie." Lies, as stated previously can be so powerful when we believe them. I have met people trapped in cages of lies. Freedom is a truth encounter.

You are not unloved simply because there are people who did not know how to love you. You are not garbage because people treated you like garbage. You are not tarnished goods just because of what you have walked through in life. **You are a gift from God**. You have infinite worth and value. If I give you a 100-dollar bill and you crumple it and smash it in the dirt, guess what? It's still worth 100 dollars. We pick that bill up, brush it off, and restore it to its previous form.

While I was in Asia, we did two different soul healing sessions, one with children who had been rescued, and the other one with women who had been rescued from human trafficking. The most powerful portion of the session with women occurred when a male on our team stepped in to repent for all the men who hurt them in their lives. We watched as women broke down, shedding tears from the depth of their souls. I recall holding one of the ladies as she sadly expressed how her parents never told her they loved her. The wounds inflicted, by not being loved by her family, opened the door for future neglect and abuse.

We want to be whole. I want you to be whole. I want to be whole. It is a journey. Maybe you will have one huge encounter with God that deals with the bulk of your pain. Maybe it will be numerous encounters, over the course of a lifetime. It's worth it to pursue healing. It's worth it to invite God into the deepest places of hurt for him to mend the broken pieces. What worked for someone else, may not be the exact path you will go through in life. Each of us has a unique story. I hope, in a future book, to reveal more of my story about overcoming.

If you need help in this area, you may reach out to Dr. Scott Bitcon (innerhealinganddeliverance.org), Dr. Charles Kraft (heartssetfrcc.org), or me (empowered-free.com). We all work with people who have been severely wounded or people who suffer from PTSD and dissociation. All of us employ faith-based tools to achieve inner healing. It is not therapy or counseling, it is a faith based prayer model that assists people in addressing their hurt with God.

I highly encourage seeking outside help for deep rooted hurt and pain. You are not alone. There are people trained to help you. Some hurt is easily healed with you and God. There are deep hurts and wounds which may require someone trained to help. There is no shame in pursuing outside help. If you have been abused, or are being abused, **seek help**. I have provided for you contact information in this chapter and in the resources section. I teach a yearly Masterclass on healing wounds of abuse. The content from that course would be another book. Therefore, I provided simple tools and resources to get you started on your journey to wellness.

Chapter 7

Beauty for Ashes
(The Restorative Power of God)

*"God, your God, will restore everything you lost;
he'll have compassion on you; he'll come back and
pick up the pieces from all the places where you
were scattered," Deuteronomy 30:3.*

Restoration, according to the dictionary, is "the action of returning something to a former owner, place, or condition."
Abuse can damage a person's sense of identity, their view of God,
their view of the church, and even shift their entire perspective to
the negative. Restoration is going into the broken places and healing the wounds. God longs to remove the broken or fractured
roots, to restore the identity and soul, and strengthen the person
who was wounded.

I understand restoration from experience with God for my own
soul. I understand on a personal level what it is like to be mistreated by people claiming to be Christians, like the following examples: to be lashed out at, to be put down, to be called a heretic,
to be sabotaged, to be yelled at/verbally abused, publicly humili-
ated, slandered, to be cursed out, word cursed from the pulpit, and
lied on. Restoration with God in several instances was quick and in
other cases it took time. I can honestly say, I stand behind inner

healing and processing all the hurt with God. My own journey has taken a longer amount of time with certain things, but other parts of the journey were quickly healed.

I firmly believe restoration of the soul causes all areas of the life to improve. I noticed I attracted better relationships and treatment once my soul was healed. I have clients who report back their marriage was restored, their relationship with God and others improved, their finances improved, their sleep improved, and they have more peace and joy. The Psalmist proclaimed in Psalm 23:3, "He refreshes and restores my soul (life)." There is new life available, new perspective available, and freedom available.

I am thankful for people who specialize in inner healing. I am eternally grateful God enters into the places that hurt and He mends the wounds on the soul. Psalm 34:18 states that God is close to the broken hearted. Job 5:11 says, "...He sets on high those who are lowly, and He lifts to safety those who mourn." The things that negatively impact us matter to God. Despite what people say about God, He does not take pleasure in the suffering of humanity. God has been misrepresented as cold, uncaring, indifferent, and unloving. God cares more than anyone about the wounds on our souls. God specializes in taking what is broken and making it new.

I will not tell you that cleaning out the wounds is always a skip in the park. There were moments of great discomfort for me, as I addressed my own negative experiences with professing Christians. Even though we are supposed to pray for people and love them, that does not mean it feels good. What I hated about the "forgive and pretend it never happened" method of dealing with mistreatment was the lack of recognition of what happened to the person mistreated. What about the restoration of the person abused or mistreated? "Oh, it sucks to be you," or "What doesn't kill you will make you stronger," were phrases directed towards those mishandled. My least favorite are the people who claim the mistreatment or abuse was to make you a stronger person.

If a natural parent subjected their child to abuse and said, "I am making you a better person," we would call Child Protective Services. Yet there are people who believe God is a child abuser. There are people who act as though God has no feelings at all or lacks compassion. There are numerous passages of the Bible that highlight the love, compassion, restoring heart, and goodness of God. God loves His children far more than we love ours (Matthew 7:11). He longs to see us restored.

There are people who misunderstand parts of the Bible and create a doctrine where abuse is allowed to thrive, which works against restoration. There can additionally be a lack of understanding of how restoration happens or awareness of the great need for restoration of the person who was abused or mistreated.

Pretending like nothing happened can be celebrated. The person who forgives and pretends they were not negatively impacted may be applauded for such strong faith. Pretending there is not an issue can create issues in the future. Part of what Jesus paid for included restoration. Part of restoration is recognizing an injury occurred. The other part is dealing with the injury.

Recall in a previous chapter I told you about the lady who lied on me, and I was publicly cursed out by people in the church because of her lies. I eventually went to our senior pastor about it, and he could not believe that being stalked by this woman and her lies was a huge deal. I could forgive. He would invite her into the office, and we would both agree that we each had a role to play in the issue. I was partially devastated that he could not see how this person's actions were not only ridiculous, they were toxic. Being in a relationship with her was like dancing in a fire with a leaky gallon of gasoline tied to my back. I never knew when she would act normal or be absolutely off the charts unstable. Why was it my responsibility to deal with her instability? It wasn't my responsibility. I set a boundary, "Do not contact me again." This woman put me through several levels of torment, and she was audacious enough to claim to be the victim.

I truly believe restoration moves beyond soul healing to accepting what happened and refusing to allow others to define how you heal from the trauma. It is traumatizing to be stalked, to have to deal with people who will not leave you alone. It is traumatizing to be in situations where you must go back to the same place where the trauma occurred. Stalking is far less traumatic, in a sense, than sexual or physical abuse, yet it's still damaging to our mental and emotional health.

I recently read a story of two teenagers who killed themselves because they suffered from survivor's guilt after a mass shooting. Even returning to the place where trauma happened can trigger trauma and post-traumatic stress. So, when we tell people, "I know that pastor molested your child, but don't leave the church," I think that is ludicrous. Every time that child returns to the surroundings where abuse happened, you are reintroducing trauma. Please don't abandon God, yet it's okay to be safe. When people say, "Oh your spouse beat you up, forgive them and go back to that place/make it work," they fail to realize what abuse actually does to the soul of a person.

There are times when restoration is removing yourself from the situation where the abuse happened. It is not always possible to heal in the place where the trauma happened. Once healed, many people can return to the place of injury and not have severe reactions.

Restoration may involve a break from trying to be strong and you seeking help. I highly recommend this to everyone, yet I have encountered people who believe that admitting they are hurting is a sign of weakness. If you break your leg, pretending it's not broken does not help you. Saying, "Wow that was awful, get me to a hospital," is wisdom. We cannot see the soul, yet soul wounds can register in the brain like physical pain. Pretending does not move us towards restoration.

I have processed numerous wounds inflicted by professing Christians and other people. Many transpired while I was very young in my faith, and a few after I had become more seasoned. The more we heal, the easier it becomes to deal with the unfortunate events that occur.

I once had a pastor call me down to the front of a church, at crowded event, to publicly embarrass me. This person was biting and rude. The person seemed to enjoy mocking me in front of other people. The person ended up being lovingly confronted by me, and they stated much of what they did was a misunderstanding and rooted in their insecurity. It did not take away their actions in front of my colleagues and friends. It did not change the negative things the person spoke over me that I and my friends had to break off. Part of my restoration in this incident was to invite God into the situation to reveal His truth. His truth did not match what the person said. I chose to believe God's truth, bless the person, and move on with my life independent of any close connection. I do not gossip about the person; I hold no ill feelings. I recognized glimmers of cruelty in the person, so I choose not to be closely linked to this person. I also let their leader know what transpired. My heart is to protect other people, not get people in trouble/be a tattle tale.

I think when we see abuse and encounter abuse/mistreatment and say nothing, it is enabling that person to move on and do the same things to others. We cannot simply pretend bad stuff is not happening. There are churches today in trouble for covering up abuse or mistreatment. When we remain silent about things that really matter, we become partners with evil.

I had a prayer team leader proclaim once, in front of everyone, that I was too broken, and a mess, and she did not have time for me. She left me standing there in front of everyone just holding my already fragile heart in my hand. Part of my restoration from this incident was to immediately go home and unpack the situation with God. I also contacted the leader of that prayer team and told them they should never allow anyone to be treated the way that person treated me. At the time, I was pretty grounded in my walk with God and was not profoundly impacted. I also know there are other people who would have been devastated to be called too broken, and too much of a mess and then just left at the altar. The person did not need to be in a position ministering to people, if she could not operate with compassion.

My biggest issue with scenarios like this one are the other Christians who watch bullying and mistreatment, and say nothing. I am prone to speaking up if I see someone picking on other people. I have lost a few relationships in my life because of pulling people aside to say, "That is not okay." I have been tagged as sensitive for not tolerating mistreatment from people.

Part of a restorative community is cultivation of safe places for people. The moment we decide to be silent, is the moment darkness wins. If you are clergy or in ministry, it's not okay to abuse people or watch abuse and do nothing. The job is to help, not harm. If we cannot help people, the least we can do is not harm them on purpose.

I have walked through restoration of my soul with God and can tell you He does restore. He will take the damage done and rebuild you stronger than you were before. Restoration is your portion.

I have encountered people on ministry teams who were supposed to train me and help, who withheld information, refused to help, and then blamed me when things did not go smoothly. I have encountered professing Christians who were friendly as long as I agreed with whatever they were teaching or believing, who later shunned me and tossed me out like rubbish.

I have been cursed, cursed from pulpits (targeted by ministers to speak death instead of life). One pastor found out I had a business. I was checking out his church, not a member. I was not serving yet, because I wanted to find out if I was supposed to be there. He got up the pulpit one Sunday and said, "Some of you here own businesses and you have not done enough for the Lord. Because you have not done enough to sow into God's Kingdom, He is going to curse you," and he looked right at me. What this pastor did not know that I was a regular giver, leading a discipleship group, running a street ministry, leading teams at the free clinic, helping orphans/widows, and planning a mission trip overseas to help with human trafficking.

I shared these experiences so you may see you are not alone. I have walked through healing with God. I learned that people are just people. **People are not primarily against you; they are for themselves.** I learned that any person not yielded to God can do horrible things to other people and either justify it or claim it's a misunderstanding. I learned that part of the restorative power of God is allowing God to give us His perspective and not to lean upon our own perspective.

What I sensed from God when I was healing from gross mistreatment from Christians was the following, "*Every person who claims me, does not know me. They have ideas about me, but they do not abide in me. People imitate what they know. People will not treat you any better than they treat me. One must abide in love, to love. I am love. In the end, I will separate out who belongs to me; the wheat from the tares. Love everyone. Use wisdom and discernment. Offer mercy and grace. Depend on my love, not the love of people. Understand that when you are sinned against, the greatest sin is against me. Every person is greatly loved by me and there are those still in process. You are in process. There are those who harm others because they hate themselves. They cannot give away love they do not possess. There are those who harm others because they have partnered with darkness; pride grips their hearts. Pride always causes damage. Some are crying out for love and attention, seeking it in the wrong places, with the wrong faces. They simply fail to abide in my Son. He is pure love. They choose to love their own way, lean to their own understanding, and act in ways they think are proper yet, they violate love. Until a person abides in my love, they cannot love themselves fully or their neighbor and especially not those they see as an enemy. My love is the key."*

Part of the restorative power of God is teaching us that **we are not victims, we are victors**. We can proclaim with assertiveness, "I am not your punching bag, not your victim. You will not continue to treat me poorly, nor anyone else on my watch." I learned that when you are kind, compassionate, and seek to honor others, it can be seen as weakness. It takes greater strength to be self-controlled and restrained than it does to be a bully and rude. It takes no strength to be hateful or dishonoring. It requires dignity and great strength to not return evil for evil.

Part of the restorative power of God is removal of all the lies spoken, the harm inflicted, and then becoming an advocate for other people. We get healed, then go help others. There are millions of people on this planet suffering in silence. There are people who come to church on Sunday, hear the sermons about submission and forgiveness, and go home to pure anguish.

God has the ability to take what was meant for harm and turn it into something good. It does not mean that abuse is good. It does <u>not</u> mean God allowed abuse or mistreatment to teach us a lesson. The abuse was not a tool so we would have a colorful story to tell. Our story can be a powerful story of hope for others. The redemptive power of God can be confused by people as His will.

Restoration involves repentance. I told you the story of our work in Asia where a teammate stood in the gap for all men. He repented on behalf of all men who hurt them. It was powerful. Have you had people from your church hurt you or shun you. On behalf of the church, I say **I am sorry for all of the hurt caused by professing Christians.** We are works in progress and claiming to be a Christian does not prevent people from sinning. Sin always hurts people. Yet there is a redeemer. His name is Jesus.

The redemption of God is powerful. There comes a point, after the daggers are removed, and the memories are healed, that a person can look back and say, "I am not happy about the abuse or mistreatment, yet I learned valuable lessons." One of the greatest lessons I learned was to pray over every relationship, every opportunity, and to not ignore red flags. I learned loving people did not mean they all had the same level of access to my life. I learned to deal with things sooner rather than later. As painful as certain situations can be, we can learn a valuable lesson that can help us or others in the future. Maybe the lesson learned is God is better than the way He is portrayed.

I would love to share with you a few of the things I learned in my process of restoration. I hope to release a more in-depth book about my walk with Jesus and the power of God to heal in the future. I hope the stories in this book help you navigate from a place of pain into a place of freedom.

People who have not suffered gross mistreatment or abuse, or do not work with abuse victims, can be clueless. They may say things that are absolutely insensitive and rude. Understand they simply cannot relate. I work with abuse victims, which increased my compassion 100 percent. There are people who struggle with empathy and compassion. They don't comprehend what empathy and compassion are and do not take the time to listen so they can understand.

God is the best person to go to with all the junk, our issues, and any pain. God can handle it all, even our anger and disappointment. You may be struggling with your trust in God or believing God. God can handle it. It may not be details or information you want to share with everyone in your church. There are people who are not qualified to counsel you. You may not wish to share your story with them in the middle of your healing process. Some may be a stumbling block to healing.

There are certain generations and people that live by the "Suck it up; deal with it," mentality. They may believe because they lived through horrific events, like the Great Depression or Vietnam, that you are being a wimp. Yes, there are things people classify as wounds that are simply offenses, yet we are not to judge the tolerance of another person. I may be unaffected by people shunning me. I am an introvert. I am often in love with books and solitude. It may impact an extrovert on a deeper level. If it makes you feel any better, when I have had the "Suck it up and deal," people in deep inner healing sessions, I have discovered some of them have a defense mechanism to shut down emotions, which is not healthy. We all have different temperaments based on our experiences in life and personalities. There are things in my life that were challenging for me, that may not be for you and vice versa.

Understand everything may not come up roses in the first round of discovery and healing. I have met a few people who became discouraged wounds were not healed in 3 hours when they have lived with them 20-50 years. It can be a journey for people. I am not stating it has to be. I am stating **if your journey takes time, it does mean you have less faith or God does not love you**. I dislike when people shame other people for not receiving breakthrough fast enough. I have heard people say, "Every person I pray for is healed, and it doesn't take all that." Then I meet people in sessions who were recipients of their ministry and their soul is deeply, deeply wounded. I wonder if the people who claim they are the superheroes of faith actually check in with people later. Restoration does not always feel like a happy experience. It can be extremely painful to allow the junk to surface, deal with the negative emotions, and move forward. Stuffing seems like a good idea until there is so much stuffing there is an explosion. Some wonder why people kill themselves, leave churches or check out. It's easy to judge and say, "They must not have had strong enough faith," or "They should have reached out." From what I have seen in my lifetime in communities of faith is dealing with emotional pain is not talked about much, grief is not talked about much, how to deal with life's tragedies in healthy ways is not talked about much. You may be expected to never complain, pretend it's all joy, and have a perpetual smile displayed on your face.

I have heard leaders say they avoid their congregants who are hurting because they don't have time to deal with hurting people. The truth is, the happy shiny people are loved and applauded. The people who push themselves to the point of breakdown and then claim it's all joy are celebrated. The people who take their masks off and claim, "This is not enjoyable, and I need help," are occasionally given a response of, "I will pray for you and here is a scripture."

My admonishment to you is to seek God and a safe community. I encourage people to go to support groups that focus on what they are walking through at the time. There is grief share. There are domestic violence survivor groups. I cultivated a group for people that is a safe community. We do not tolerate abuse, mistreatment, or putting others down because they are struggling. I also have asked God over the years to place safe people in my life.

I can tell you that inviting God into the places that hurt and continuing with inner healing does get easier. You do develop strength and learn to rely on God's strength. You can be healed to the point where a memory no longer controls you with pain. It is possible; I have piles of testimonials from soul healing sessions with people to validate that claim.

God has no intention of leaving us in a place of pain and torment or as a pile of ashes. He promises beauty for ashes, joy for mourning, and double honor for former shame. God loves to make things better than before they were broken. Yes, it's a process for many. It is worth the journey.

I would not be writing to you if there was not restorative power in God. There were moments in my walk with God where I wanted nothing to do with church people. Other than my parents, I had seen enough to make me never want to go to church. My heart was restored. I realized every single person is a work in progress and every person attending church is not a true Christian.

We can choose to be the change we want to see in the world. Part of restoration is seeing how we can be part of the solutions. We can come in and be an example, refuse to tolerate bad teaching on submission and misrepresentation of Jesus. We can be a voice for the voiceless. We can say no, not on my watch. We can take a stance against violence, abuse, mistreatment and be an advocate for those still hurting.

I am praying for you right now, as I type, that you will be restored fully! God loves you profoundly. Your wounding is not your identity. **You are a VICTOR**! You were born to live victorious. You may have been victimized; you do not have to stay victimized.

Chapter 8

From Victim to Victor!

"Perseverance and perspective until victory"
-Lincoln Diaz-Balart.

You made it to chapter 8! I planned to write seven chapters, then added an additional chapter on boundaries. I hope at this point you are overflowing with hope. I am praying for you. As I type I am praying that your heart and soul are healed. I am praying that you are saturated with a profound understanding that God cares about you! I am so sorry that there are people who claimed to love Jesus who hurt you, abused you, abused your children, mistreated you, shunned you, talked about you, gossiped, lied, stalked you, or put you down. I am sorry if you were treated as though you had no value, because **you have tremendous value**. The value of something is determined by how much a person is willing to pay for it, and Jesus paid for you with His life. God loves you with an everlasting love.

Part of moving from a victim to a victor is finding identity in who God says we are and not how people treat us. I saw a quote that I loved. It said, "You are upset about not being loved by people who don't even love themselves. You are allowing people to tell you who you are, and they don't even know who they are." I will say it over and over that a person who does not love themselves cannot love you and people imitate the God they envision in their minds.

It would be wonderful if people loved us the way God loves us. It requires a yielded life to God and first receiving God's love. There are people who spend their entire lives going to church and they have no real depth in their relationship with God. We are transformed not by our church attendance, but by our relationship with God.

Victims can see their situation as hopeless and their lives as powerless. **Victors see themselves as powerful**. Maybe as a child you were helpless, but you are not helpless today. There is always hope in Jesus. Hope is an expectation of good. I love one of phrases I heard from Bill Johnson, he stated, "Any place we are without hope is under the influence of a lie." God is full of hope. When we feel hopeless, He loves to share His hope with us. When we feel weak and without strength, God loves to share His strength with us. When we are beyond tired of the drama and trauma, there is comfort available in God. I encourage people not to give up on God even if they are fed-up with Christians. Hey, even Jesus escaped to just be alone with the Father.

Victors see the possibility to turn pain into power. I cannot change the way I was treated by certain clergy, leaders, or people in the church. I can choose not to be like them and set a better example. There are people who taught me what not to do if I were ever given more responsibility or influence. In my family, we were taught to treat the CEO and janitor with the same respect. I learned from the people who put me on blast (slang phrase for attempts to publicly humiliate me), that insecurity is toxic. Insecure people seek to denigrate others. I can use what was intended to cause me to shrink back to propel me forward.

Your story can be a tool for growth and inspiration for those who have a similar story. It's incredible to see others overcome and emerge powerfully on the other side of challenges. When we have the knowledge of how to overcome, we can speak, teach, and influence from experience and not secondhand information.

I have encountered numerous people in my walk who were much more comfortable receiving ministry from a person who understood how to help abuse victims. I have hugged and wiped tears from people who have pastors who are too busy and are not interested in the hurt of abuse victims. I have had conversations with people who were bullied into staying in abusive friendships and marriages who were relieved when they discovered that they were not irrational for wanting to set limits or even get to a safe place. I have received messages from people who were thankful for teachings about what godly submission is and what it's not. I have additionally received gratitude from people for teachings shared on how the word submission has been twisted to mean something it was never intended to mean.

God can take even the most devastating things and use them as tools to help others, propel us forward, and give us hope when things seem bleak. There is a blessing on the other side.

Walking through being greatly wounded by Christians and healed by God gives us a perspective of God we may not have had before. I learned that God is far more interested in loving me than turning me into the clone of Jesus. God is far more concerned with the condition of our hearts than our performance. I learned that though God loves gratitude, He is not fond of fake Christianity. "I know our dog died, our house burned to the ground, and my spouse left me, but I am rejoicing in the Lord!" **God loves authenticity**. "Hey God, I miss my dog. I wish my house was not a pile of ashes, and the timing of my spouse leaving is less than ideal." That was my made-up scenario, yet I have had several instances in my life where it was just one deluge of bad news after another. As I write this to you, we have had three deaths in our family in the past 5 months, 2 within the past 2 weeks. Have I been leaping around my house singing, "God is good all the time?" Well no. There have been days where it has been, "Okay God, I need your strength today. I love you. I am ready for relief." I am pretty real with God. He already knows what we truly feel anyway. God is authentic. God is not inviting us into fake Christianity.

Being a victor does not mean we will feel like Superman or Wonder Woman every day. It does not mean we will trust Christians easily again either. It may take time to warm up to new people or trust again. This is normal. I have heard the wackiest things from people about trust. One person said, "Love believes the best of everyone." Okay, then post your social security number or credit card number online. You are not willing to do that right? Why? Because there are people with great motives and those with bad motives. God encourages us to love and seek to believe the best, that does not mean be foolish and lack wisdom. Wisdom is learning to examine who people really are before we give them VIP access to our life.

We can learn from what we go through and teach those lessons we have learned to others. They may not always want to listen, yet we can try. I try to teach young women red flags on abuse. I disciple and mentor. I put information and articles online that address many of the topics in the book and more. You can too. Please don't allow abuse to be the final chapter of your story or the theme of your life. **We are not what we have been through; we are who God says we are**. A horrible chapter is not the entire book. If you see patterns of abuse or mistreatment, start inviting God into your soul to heal the wounds.

I admire people who have walked through the fire and emerged alive. I love the stories of people who could have laid down and died, proclaimed perpetual victimhood, but they refused to die.

They got knocked down, but they got back up again. My heart is crying out for you and every victim of abuse. **You can get back up again!** Your story does not end here. There is a warrior inside of you who will emerge. The journey may not be skipping through roses every day, yet if you commit to show up each day, I think you will begin to see roses emerging from the thorns. As long as you are still breathing, there is more story to be written. Your best days can be ahead of you. Redemption and restoration are your portion!

Eventually you learn to put a fence around your heart, not a wall. Therefore, people can see your heart, but only those invited can come inside. You learn to spot the people with matches and gasoline and let them know your house (soul) is not their next burn down project. You learn to establish boundaries and pray over every relationship. You begin to ask God for insight on who is a divine connection and who should just be an associate. You learn your value and worth on a much greater level. Most of all you learn empathy.

I am cheering for you. I believe in you. More than believing in you, I trust in the God who has walked me through the most challenging seasons of my life. Even in moments when I felt forsaken, there was love. He stood there in love, over and over picking up the pieces, sometimes apologizing on behalf of those who created the devastation. He is the one who has repeatedly stood in the field of ashes stating, "I will rebuild. Better than before."

Our mindset needs to align with victory. After we walk through inviting God to sift through the ruins of our soul, we simply must align our thoughts to a new way of thinking. **"I am not a victim anymore. I am empowered by God to live above what was done to me."** My prayer is that our minds are cleansed of every lie and fortified by God's truth. As stated repeatedly, dealing with the wounds on the soul brings healing. I can believe I can run a marathon, yet if my leg is broken I am most likely not going to run. Soul healing is dealing with the broken parts so we can run.

Freedom is available. Victory is available. We each have a unique destiny and purpose. A person's life should not be sidelined by abuse and mistreatment. Yes, it happened. I am so sorry for any abuse or mistreatment. It can be healed. I have seen people who have the worst abuse stories who are walking in freedom today. There were moments or seasons of hopelessness, then they stepped into healing. They stopped hiding. They ceased pretending. They acknowledged the pain and invited God into the painful situations. It's your turn!

I am believing God for your healing. I am believing for all the pain to be released and healed. I am believing for complete victory from the haunting of painful memories. I hope your perspective of who you are and who God is shifts to the positive. If you are reading this, you survived and now it is time to thrive. During abuse, defense mechanisms can kick in to keep a person alive. We were never intended to live in perpetual survival mode. We were created to be overcomers, conquerors, and victors.

I am speaking life over you!

I declare:

You are not what happened to you.

You are loved, intensely loved by God.

Your life is highly valuable.

Your life is a gift!

You are a victor not a victim.

You will overcome.

The best days are ahead and not behind you.

You are an overcomer!

You are powerful, not helpless.

You are not how people treated you.

You may shift these declarations to I am!

I am not what happened to me.

I am loved, greatly loved by God.

My life is highly valuable.

My life is a gift!

I am a victor not a victim.

I will overcome.

The best days are ahead and not behind me.

I am an overcomer!

I am powerful, not helpless.

I am not how people treated me.

I highly recommend to speak life over yourself. We begin to believe what we repeatedly hear. You may want to write out these declarations on a card or your mirror and say them often. Victorious living is linked to a healthy mind. If negative thoughts arise, one exercise you can do is write them out. Negative in our head looks different when we write them out. Another exercise you can do it just start speaking out what you see in the room. "The carpet is beige. The sky is blue." It helps move the mind away from the negative thoughts. If a memory continues to resurface, invite God into that memory. "God, I invite you into the memories that haunt me. I invite healing." Once again, this may require another trained person, especially if there is dissociation (deep fractures in the personality).

God believes in you. I am believing for you to walk in the fullness of all Jesus died to give you. Your portion is abundance, health, and a sound mind. It is not abuse, torment, and a life of oppression. Will you join me in prayer?

God, I want to be whole. I speak to every part of me that I want to be healed and whole. I invite you God into my soul to heal me completely. I want to walk in the fullness of all you payed for in Jesus. I release all my pain to you God. I release all the pain, trauma, hurt, offense, unforgiveness, and woundedness. I do not want to carry it anymore. I am destined to walk in victory! I was created to be an overcomer. I am not what happened to me. I ask you to help those who hurt me to know you and truly know what love is. Fill us with your unfailing love.

Never forget, you are profoundly loved!

Key Terms and Concepts

Abuse: A violation of another person which involves mistreatment, cruelty, or misuse. Abuse may be physical, emotional, verbal, sexual, spiritual, or express itself in control and/or manipulation.

Dissociation: the disconnection or separation of something from something else or the state of being disconnected. Separation of normally related mental processes, resulting in one group functioning independently from the rest, leading in extreme cases to disorders such as multiple personality.[1]

[Dissociation is a disconnection between a person's thoughts, memories, feelings, actions or sense of who he or she is. This is a normal process that everyone has experienced. Examples of mild, common dissociation include daydreaming, highway hypnosis or "getting lost" in a book or movie, all of which involve "losing touch" with awareness of one's immediate surroundings.

During a traumatic experience such as an accident, disaster or crime victimization, dissociation can help a person tolerate what might otherwise be too difficult to bear. In situations like these, a person may dissociate the memory of the place, circumstances or feelings about the overwhelming event, mentally escaping from the fear, pain and horror. This may make it difficult to later remember

---

[1] Dictionary Definition

the details of the experience, as reported by many disaster and accident survivors.][2]

Post-Traumatic Stress Disorder: a condition of persistent mental and emotional stress occurring as a result of injury or severe psychological shock, typically involving disturbance of sleep and constant vivid recall of the experience, with dulled responses to others and to the outside world.[1]

Soul: The soul is comprised of the mind, will, and emotions. It is not the same as the spirit.

[While the two words (soul and spirit) are often used interchangeably, the primary distinction between soul and spirit in man is that the soul is the animate life, or the seat of the senses, desires, affections, and appetites. The spirit is that part of us that connects, or refuses to connect, to God. Our spirits relate to His Spirit, either accepting His promptings and conviction, thereby proving that we belong to Him (Romans 8:16) or resisting Him and proving that we do not have spiritual life (Acts 7:51).][3]

---

[2] https://www.psychiatry.org/patients-families/dissociative-disorders/what-are-dissociative-disorders

[3] https://www.compellingtruth.org/difference-soul-spirit.html

Bonus Content

Seen by God (Poem)

I see you in the ashes,

carrying sadness, grief, and shame.

I see you hurting,

and I long to take away your pain.

This is not your final story.

This is not the end.

I will transform those scars,

into beauty again.

I see you in the ashes,

questioning your value and your worth.

I see you looking for answers,

and searching for hope.

I see you,

and I love you.

Right here,

right where you are,

there I am.

You are never alone.

Though it may seem I was far away,

I was with you.

I was weeping.

I was crying out for you.

I see the ashes,

and long to give you beauty.

My heart desires to give you

dancing for mourning,

joy for sorrow,

double honor for your shame,

and for you to participate in the divine exchange.

Trade torment for peace.

Trade pain for healing.

Trade with Me.

Reach out your hand to Me.

I want to exchange your pain for My promises.

I want your latter to be better than your former.

I want to love you past your moments of pain.

I long to walk down the halls of your heart,

and remove the marks of abuse, hurt, or shame.

I long to paint My murals there,

of everlasting love and grace.

My grace empowers you to live victorious.

You were created to live abundantly.

Come to Me.

Find life and restoration in Me.

I am not against you.

I am for you.

There is nothing you can do to make me love you more.

There is nothing you can do to make me love you less.

I love you.

I have always loved you.

I have not blocked all pain.

I have opened My heart to see you made whole.

I will not force My will on anyone,

therefore, there is evil in your world.

Humanity does not choose as I would choose,

and there are casualties which breaks My heart.

I see you.

I see you struggle to find Me in your pain.

I see the lies that try to convince you,

that I delight in human suffering.

I delight in you knowing how much I love you.

I delight in your laughter.

I delight in you knowing who you truly are.

I do not delight in your suffering or your pain.

I see you,

and I want you.

I want to know you and for you to know My heart.

I am with you on your best days.

I am with you on your worst days.

I am with you through it all.

You can call on My name.

You can cry out for comfort, help, and love.

I will answer.

I will come running,

with arms overflowing with love.

I love you.

I will always love you.

My beloved,

you are not alone.

About the Author

Erin Lamb loves to empower others and see them fulfill their divine destiny. Part of her training is in research and development, science, and engineering. She is also trained in deep inner healing to assist those who suffer from PTSD and dissociation using faith-based methods. Her program has helped numerous people and receives A+ ratings. Yearly the Deep Inner Healing Masterclass trains people to help victims of severe abuse.

She is the author of I Thought I Knew What Love Was and Confident & Free, the founder and CEO of Lamb Enterprises LLC, and Operation God is Love. Lamb Enterprises specializes in coaching, mentoring, teaching, masterclasses on wholeness, publishing, and digital creation. Operation God is Love (OGL) is a not for profit initiative which serves the least, last, and lost in the community. It includes homeless outreach, free clinic support, and overseas missions. Recently OGL served in Cambodia with women and children rescued or in need of rescue from human trafficking.

Websites:

Business: https://www.empowered-free.com
Ministry: http://www.OperationGodisLove.org
Blog: http://www.Ithoughtiknewwhatlovewas.com

Recommended Resources

Books

2 Hours to Freedom (Deep Inner Healing) by Dr. Charles Kraft

Why Not Women (Covers Paul's Letters/Wrong Teachings on Submission) by Loren Cunningham and David Joel Hamilton

Without Rival by Lisa Bevere

Soul Decrees by Katie Souza

Breaking Free by Beth Moore

Battlefield of the Mind by Joyce Meyer

For Abuse Victims or to Report Abuse

The National Domestic Violence Hotline:
https://www.thehotline.org/
1-800-799-7233 (1-800-787-3224 (TTY))

National Sexual Assault Hotline: https://rainn.org/about-national-sexual-assualt-telephone-hotline
1-800-656-HOPE (4673)

National Human Trafficking Hotline: humantraffickinghotline.org
1 (888) 373-7888
Text (sms): 233733